The Licensing Exam Review Guide in Nursing Home Administration

James E. Allen, PhD, MSPH, NHA, IP, is an associate professor of Health Policy and Administration Emeritus at the University of North Carolina at Chapel Hill and president of LongTermCareEducation.com, a national resource website for information on the long-term care field. He has 30-plus years of experience in teaching and conducting research in the field of health care administration. He taught courses at the University of North Carolina at Chapel Hill in long-term care administration, medical ethics, and the organization and financing of health care delivery in the United States. He has provided legal consultation in long-term care litigation matters across 10 states.

The website www.longtermcareedu.com (or www.ltce.com) provides more than 500 pages of state-by-state, up-to-date information on such subjects as:

- Becoming a nursing home administrator
- Becoming an assisted living administrator
- Exploring a career in long-term care
- Contacting the state licensing authority in each state
- Enrolling in college programs in each state
- Obtaining key publications in the long-term care field
- Getting continuing education units.

Dr. Allen can be reached via e-mail through the website, or directly at jeallen@mindspring.com or jamesallen@unc.edu, or via phone (1-929-815-0387) or fax (1-919-953-6825). Continuing education units for both nursing home and assisted living administrators are also available through the website (www .LongTermCareEducation.com).

Additional resources from Springer Publishing Company are available to persons preparing to become long-term care administrators:

Nursing Home Federal Requirements and Guidelines to Surveyors, Eighth Edition: A user-friendly rendering of the Centers for Medicare and Medicaid Services nursing home inspection requirements.

Nursing Home Administration, Seventh Edition: The definitive textbook of essential knowledge for obtaining licensure and employment as a nursing home administrator.

Visit www.springerpub.com for more information

The Licensing Exam Review Guide in Nursing Home Administration

Seventh Edition

James E. Allen, PhD, MSPH, NHA, IP

SPRINGER PUBLISHING COMPANY
NEW YORK

Springer Publishing Company, LLC
11 West 42nd Street
New York, NY 10036
www.springerpub.com

Acquisitions Editor: Sheri W. Sussman
Composition: Newgen KnowledgeWorks

ISBN: 978-0-8261-2918-5
e-book ISBN: 978-0-8261-2919-2

15 16 17 18 / 5 4 3 2 1

The author and the publisher of this Work have made every effort to use sources believed to be reliable to provide information that is accurate and compatible with the standards generally accepted at the time of publication. The author and publisher shall not be liable for any special, consequential, or exemplary damages resulting, in whole or in part, from the readers' use of, or reliance on, the information contained in this book. The publisher has no responsibility for the persistence or accuracy of URLs for external or third-party Internet websites referred to in this publication and does not guarantee that any content on such websites is, or will remain, accurate or appropriate.

Library of Congress Cataloging-in-Publication Data
Allen, James E. (James Elmore), 1935- , author.
  The licensing exam review guide in nursing home administration / James E. Allen. — Seventh edition.
    p. ; cm.
  Includes bibliographical references and index.
  ISBN 978-0-8261-2918-5 — ISBN 978-0-8261-2919-2 (e-book)
  I. Title.
  [DNLM: 1. Nursing Homes—organization & administration--United States—Examination Questions.
2. Long-Term Care—organization & administration—United States—Examination Questions. WX 18.2]
  RA999.A35
  362.16068—dc23   2015033677

Special discounts on bulk quantities of our books are available to corporations, professional associations, pharmaceutical companies, health care organizations, and other qualifying groups. If you are interested in a custom book, including chapters from more than one of our titles, we can provide that service as well.

For details, please contact:
Special Sales Department, Springer Publishing Company, LLC
11 West 42nd Street, 15th Floor, New York, NY 10036–8002
Phone: 877–687-7476 or 212–431-4370; Fax: 212–941-7842
E-mail: sales@springerpub.com

Printed in the United States of America by Bradford & Bigelow.

Contents

---

*Numbering of headings in this Review Guide corresponds to key headings in *Nursing Home
Administration*, Seventh Edition.

Introduction: Uses of This Study Guide for the NAB Domains of Practice

The review questions in this guide are intended for use by persons who are studying for the national licensure examination.

Sample study questions are provided from several texts and sources in the long-term care field, including more than 70 questions on the Final Rules for Medicare and Medicaid Requirements for Long-Term Care Facilities: Federal Appendix PP and Nurse's Aide Training and Competency Evaluation Programs.

National examination questions are picked by computer from a bank of more than 2,000 items. On average, more than 3,000 persons take this examination each year. Generally, about three unique exams are offered each year. The National Association of Boards of Examiners for Long-Term Care Administrators (NAB) exam is taken on a computer and each time the exam is taken, the applicant will have a different set of questions unique to that exam.

Format of the National Exam

The national examination is set up in the multiple-choice, one-best-answer style of question to test the level of each candidate's knowledge.

This review guide is designed to acquaint the user with relevant terms and provide practice in the multiple-choice, one-best-answer examination format.

Two basic benefits are received: (a) feedback on comprehension of the terms and concepts in areas similar to those covered in the national examination, and (b) experience with the multiple-choice testing format used in the national exam.

Use of this review guide without the text book, *Nursing Home Administration*, Seventh Edition, and other similar sources achieves only initial knowledge about the field of nursing home administration. The bits and pieces of information obtained from these study questions are not a substitute for systematically studying the basic principles and information contained in the reading materials for Long Term Care Education (LTCE) 201 and 202 (www.LongTermCareEducation.com) and other equivalent resources.

The "One-Best-Answer"
Testing Format

There is always one best answer to each of the questions in this book and on the exam. In the following question, only one answer can be correct.

> The Lifespan Respite Care Act, allowing for the first time public payment to relatives to give care to family members, was passed in _____.
> 1. 1995
> 2. 2006
> 3. 2007
> 4. 2008

Because the Lifespan Respite Care Act was passed in 2006 (answer 2) all of the other answers are completely wrong.

In the following question, however, options 1, 2, and 4 are all partially correct, but 3 is the correct answer because it is the most complete (best) answer.

> In the nursing facility a resident may perform services for the facility if the services are _____.
> 1. Voluntary
> 2. Paid at or above prevailing rates
> 3. In the plan of care
> 4. Light duty in nature

All four options are partially correct; services performed must be voluntarily assumed, paid for at or above prevailing wage rates, and light duty in nature. However, even if services performed by a resident meet the three requirements in options 1, 2, and 4, they are prohibited if not in the resident's plan of care. Hence, 3 is the one best answer.

Following is an additional example.

> Control is the evaluation by the organization decision makers of _____.
> 1. Capital assets
> 2. The outputs of the organization
> 3. Deficit spending
> 4. Employee goals

The correct answer is 2, the outputs of the organization. Each of the other options is potentially correct. Organization decision makers *do* evaluate or make managerial judgments about capital assets, deficit spending if it occurs, and employee goals.

However, the keyword in the question is *control.* The correct answer is the answer that best defines control behavior by organizational decision makers. Answer 2 more fully defines control than any of the other three.

Sometimes the respondent is asked to mark the answer that is the least correct. For example,

The National Labor Relations Board does not _____.
1. Determine what the bargaining units shall be
2. Conduct representation elections by secret ballot
3. Investigate unfair labor practices
4. Make court decisions

The answer is 4. Answers 1, 2, and 3 are all activities the National Labor Relations Board *does do.*

Deciding What the Question Is

A key to successfully answering multiple-choice questions is correctly deciding what is being asked. For example:

> In states that still require government permission to build new nursing homes, if the health authority believes a shortage of beds exists, it may _____.
> 1. Require that additional beds be built
> 2. Let a contract for building new beds
> 3. Advertise for bids
> 4. Issue a permit to build (Certificate of Need)

The issue being tested here is: Does the respondent know the functions and typical scope of powers exercised by a public health planning authority? The respondent needs to know that powers of health planning authorities are limited to granting permission for the applicant to build new beds.

To answer the question correctly, the respondent needs to further understand that local and state health planning authorities normally have no power to require that additional beds be built, to let contracts for building new beds, or to advertise for or let bids for constructing facilities with new beds. These are activities performed by the owners of the new facilities.

Deciding What the Answer Is

Once the respondent has accurately decided *the question* about which he or she is being tested, the *one best answer* to the question must be selected. If the respondent knows what the answer ought to be, a useful technique is to look immediately for the correct answer. For example,

> For nursing facilities, meeting accreditation requirements set by the JCAHO (Joint Commission on Accreditation for Healthcare Organizations) is _____.
>
> 1. Voluntary
> 2. Mandatory
> 3. Required to receive Medicaid payments
> 4. Required to receive Medicare payments

If the reader knows that meeting requirements set by JCAHO are entirely voluntary for nursing facilities, he or she should look immediately for the correct answer, which in this case is 1. The other options can then be read to ensure that there is not a better or more correct or complete option to mark as the correct answer.

To answer this question correctly, the reader needs specific information; for example, knowledge of Medicare and Medicaid requirements for nursing facilities and the federal requirements that must be met for reimbursement for Medicare or Medicaid patient charges. If read hastily, this question could be deceptive because *hospital* accreditation by JCAHO *is* required for hospital eligibility for reimbursement of Medicare patient charges. The equivalent for nursing homes is to meet the federal requirements set by the federal and state governments.

Thus, several areas of understanding may be tested simultaneously by a single question such as the one in the example.

Strategies for Test Taking

Test taking, like driving a car, is an acquired skill. It is a complex task that, once learned, can become second nature when the techniques are established. In addition, practice in answering the types of questions that may be asked can ease the tension level when in the actual test situation. Following are some strategies for taking computer-based multiple-choice tests.

In an examination consisting of 150 questions, each with four possible answers, the reader must cycle through 600 possible answers. Giving equal energy to each of the 600 possible options can lead to mental fatigue early in the examination and may result in unintentional errors. Several *techniques* are available *to help reduce mental fatigue.*

MARKING QUESTIONS FOR LATER REVIEW

The test will contain questions that the reader can answer with confidence, but there will inevitably be questions where the answer is only a guess.

To save time and energy, it is advisable to proceed through the entire exam at a steady pace, marking for later review questions about which the reader is unsure.

Do not try to puzzle out each doubtful or unknown question in the order in which it appears. Go on to the next. This ensures reasonably quick progress through the exam. Using this strategy, it will be found that a large proportion of questions will have been correctly answered during the first run through. A second attempt to complete the remaining items will often reveal the answers at this stage.

MAKING FINAL CHOICES

Once all items have been marked, it is time for a second run through for a final decision about the choices made.

Experience has shown that the first answer chosen is often the best one. However, if the respondent is sure, on restudying the question, that a different response is the correct one, the answer originally marked should be changed.

USING THE TIME AVAILABLE

The goal is to achieve the best possible score on the examination. For most people this should mean taking advantage of all of the time available. Rereading the questions and assuring oneself that the correct answer has been chosen is usually time well spent. In multiple-choice questions, there is often *one keyword or phrase* that may elude the reader on the first reading, but might change the answer dramatically.

FINAL REVIEW

If there is time, the respondent should assure himself or herself that the *question being asked* in every item has been correctly understood and the correct answer marked.

NAB Domain: Management, Governance, and Leadership

Learning How to Manage the Health Care Organization

Questions 1 to 31 portray often-encountered situations in the nursing home profession. The answers and rationale to Questions 1 to 31 can be found in the section of this book preceding the Answer Key.

Question 32 to the end flow sequentially through the topics in *Nursing Home Administration*, Seventh Edition, by James E. Allen, PhD, MSPH, NHA, IP. Answers can be found in the textbook on the page numbers in parentheses following each of these questions. In Part 6, answers can be found in *Nursing Home Administration*, Seventh Edition, and *Nursing Home Federal Requirements: Guidelines to Surveyors and Survey Protocols*, Eighth Edition, by James E. Allen, MSPH, PhD, NHA, IP (both published by Springer Publishing Company). Those found in *Nursing Home Federal Requirements* are distinguished by the reference "(See Federal Requirements)."

---

1. The most likely single cause for the series of bankruptcies among larger nursing home chains around the year 2000 was ____.
   1. Too small increases in government reimbursement rates
   2. Paying too much for acquisitions in 1998 and 1999
   3. Not taking advantage of falling interest rates
   4. Thinking too small

2. In a chance conversation with the owner of an eight-facility chain, the newly hired administrator for the oldest facility in the chain indicates that, because the mortgage is fully retired, the administrator will concentrate more on being effective than efficient since the Quality Indicators are all at or above the state's average. The owner would likely ____.
   1. Be pleased
   2. Be distressed
   3. Be content
   4. Praise the newly hired administrator

3. Occupancy of Facility A has been a steady 70% since the Prospective Payment System was introduced. Two weeks ago, a new 120-bed, equally equipped facility opened several blocks away. The Facility A administrator tells the admissions counselor to continue the usual recruitment approach. The chain owners ought to _____.
   1. Rest comfortably
   2. Seek a new administrator
   3. Appoint a new admissions counselor
   4. Take no action

4. Bankruptcies among larger nursing home chains prior to 2000 _____.
   1. Were frequent
   2. Were ubiquitous
   3. Were highly unusual
   4. Were routinely declared to avoid too much accumulated debt

5. Under the Prospective Payment System, nursing facilities' reimbursed costs _____.
   1. Were about the same as previously
   2. Were more bundled
   3. Used an unbundled cost structure
   4. Were reimbursement for actual costs

6. In recent years, Medicare has _____.
   1. Allowed facilities to make a modest profit
   2. Shifted more costs onto nursing facilities
   3. Eased up on economic pressures previously placed on facilities
   4. Remained relatively unchanged in its reimbursement structure

7. The nurse newly promoted to director of nursing insists on giving four RN hours of patient care each day on the Alzheimer's wing in the 175-bed facility. The administrator should _____.
   1. Praise the new director of nursing for her resident centeredness
   2. Appoint an assistant director of nursing
   3. Adapt the job description to fit her pattern
   4. Seek a new director of nursing

8. The applicant for the administrator position in a facility near a large teaching hospital insists that, as before in his rural facility, if hied he would not let the Medicare reimbursement policies affect his case mix. This applicant _____.
   1. Should be hired
   2. Is likely to succeed if hired
   3. Can likely succeed in his goal
   4. Is out of touch

9. The newly hired assistant to the administrator insists that the organizational chart dotted line between this position and the Department of Nursing be a solid line. The administrator should _____.
   1. Agree in general
   2. Agree to this special case
   3. Ask the director of nursing for his or her opinion
   4. Be forewarned

10. The medical supplies provider tells the administrator of a facility that has not paid bills for the past 3 months but is now operating under a bankruptcy judge's approved plan for restructuring, that no more deliveries will be made until past bills are fully paid. The medical supplies provider _____.
    1. Is smart to cut losses at that point
    2. Does not understand how bankruptcy works
    3. Will now likely get his past due bills paid
    4. Is farsighted

11. An administrator who adopts the leadership-by-walking-around (LBWA) approach by walking through the facility weekly and intently observing has _____.
    1. Become an effective leader
    2. Chosen a good management style
    3. Failed to understand LBWA
    4. Implemented a useful strategy

12. The nursing facility administrator who, using the leadership-by-walking around (LBWA) technique, succeeds in actually making appropriate corrections on the spot during her rounds _____.
    1. Is effectively implementing the concept
    2. Gains additional power through the process
    3. Exhibits appropriate leadership
    4. Does not understand LBWA

13. The rate of increase in the total number of nursing facilities in the United States during the years 2008 to 2012 is _____.
    1. Likely to be about level
    2. Likely to double
    3. Likely to triple to accommodate the baby boomer generation
    4. Likely to decrease markedly

14. The applicant for administrator of the facility insists that he has successfully used democratic leadership to the exclusion of all other leadership styles. The interviewer should _____.
    1. Recommend hiring this candidate
    2. Praise the candidate
    3. Be favorably impressed
    4. Continue to interview candidates

15. The candidate for administrator said that she used a variety of administrative styles, but could not say exactly which she would use in every circumstance. The interviewer should be _____.
1. Favorably impressed
2. Unfavorably impressed
3. Concerned about possible indecisiveness
4. Looking for one leadership style

16. The candidate for administrator indicated that he consistently chose the charismatic style of leadership. This should _____ the interviewer.
1. Reassure
2. Alert
3. Confirm the candidate's qualifications to
4. Please

17. The costs of providing subacute care to nursing home residents _____.
1. Is perhaps triple that of the more typical patient
2. Covered by Medicare
3. Absorbed by Medicaid if Medicare coverage is inadequate
4. Mostly covered by private insurance

18. The nurse supervisor who had just been appointed director of nursing announced at the first department head meeting that she had circulated a memo among the nurses that only formal communications were to be allowed in the nursing department. The administrator should _____.
1. Be relieved
2. Confirm the decision
3. Be supportive
4. Anticipate problems

19. The department head was not surprised to learn that an employee had heard only the positive comments to the employee and ignored the criticisms. The department head's grasp of the communication process is _____.
1. Deficient
2. Appropriate
3. Out of focus
4. Inadequate

20. The administrator routinely accepted as a nearly exclusive information source the director of nursing's positive reports that nursing was going well. The administrator is _____.
1. Showing appropriate confidence in the director of nursing
2. Utilizing the director of nursing properly
3. Realizing a successful appointment has been made
4. Placing himself at risk

21. Periodic shortage of nurses available for nursing home employment _____.
    1. Is being solved by community college programs
    2. Is decreasing
    3. Can be readily solved by hiring temporary nurses
    4. Is likely to remain for the foreseeable future

22. Congress and the federal rule makers behave as if the facility will run successfully if Congress and the Centers for Medicare and Medicaid Services can write enough rules. They are _____.
    1. Incorrect
    2. Correct, according to behavior theory
    3. Pessimistic about the need for rules
    4. Correct, according to emerging management theory

23. When the administrator notices that the director of nursing seeks to turn as many duties as possible over to housekeeping, the administrator should conclude that the director of nursing is _____.
    1. Behaving normally
    2. Holding a grudge against housekeeping
    3. Unwilling to be cooperative
    4. Wielding power desirably

24. The administrator insists that a timely copy of all reports generated within the facility come across her desk before anyone signs them. The administrator is _____.
    1. Not rationalizing her management information system
    2. Making appropriate and desirable requests
    3. Exercising good judgment
    4. Initiating an appropriate management information system

25. The administrator notices that incident reports are being insufficiently filled out, but does nothing, believing that the situation will likely correct itself. The administrator is _____.
    1. Practicing effective control
    2. Likely to be correct
    3. Failing to control effectively
    4. Right to monitor the situation for a period of time

26. Corporate sends a directive to its flagship facility administrator directing the administrator's attention more toward the outcome of resident care than the cost of resident care during the coming 12 months. Corporate is more concerned with _____ than with _____.
    1. Effectiveness; efficiency
    2. Efficiency; effectiveness
    3. Expenses/inputs
    4. Expenses/throughput

27. The long-term care sector receiving increased funding and attention from the federal government is the _____.
    1. Home health care sector
    2. Volunteer hospice group association
    3. Long-term care hospital sector
    4. Private insurance industry

28. The concept that nursing homes should be reimbursed by states for their actual costs was part of the _____.
    1. Emerging Medicare approach
    2. Federal administration's goal as seen in new budgetary appropriations
    3. Hatch Amendment
    4. Goal statements of most state governments

29. The intense health care cost-shifting efforts among providers such as Medicare, Medicaid, and local governments are _____.
    1. On the wane
    2. Likely to continue
    3. Leading to increased reimbursements
    4. Good for the nursing home profession

30. Worried about the level of actual resident care being achieved in the facility, the administrator directs the nurses to spend less time charting and more time focusing on the effectiveness of care being given to residents. The likely result will be _____.
    1. Better resident care, possibly increased deficiency citations
    2. Better resident care, decreased deficiency citations
    3. No real improvement in resident care, decreased charting
    4. Greater sensitivity to residents' needs and better documentation

31. The new social worker informs the head of nursing that admissions is all she has time for and that nursing must monitor and document each resident's sociopsychological experiences. The new social worker is _____.
    1. Responding appropriately to priorities
    2. Achieving a better balance of assignments within the facility
    3. Responding inappropriately
    4. Likely to improve the case mix dramatically

1.1 MANAGEMENT FUNCTIONS*

32. Today the twin forces of _____ and _____ are revolutionizing the delivery of health care. (*p. 2*)
    1. Technology/patient rights
    2. Obamacare/patient data legislation
    3. Technology/patient data legislation
    4. New inventions/rapid adoption of inventions

---

*Answers can be found in *Nursing Home Administration*, Seventh Edition, on the page numbers in parentheses following each question.

33. Most of the multiple new devices to monitor and diagnose each individual's health status are creating new monitoring and diagnostic capacities _____. (p. 2)
    1. Outside the hospital
    2. Outside the doctor's office
    3. Outside the hospital and doctors office
    4. Primarily within the hospital setting

34. For the nursing facility setting, the new capacities to monitor residents' health offer dramatic new opportunities to improve _____. (p. 2)
    1. Diabetes treatment
    2. Pneumonia management
    3. Infection control techniques
    4. Chronic disease management

35. Patient data legislation, such as the most recent health care legislation, has set into motion a nationwide policy to promote patients' access to their _____. (p. 2)
    1. Rights
    2. Personal data
    3. Medical records
    4. Family history

36. Under the Affordable Care Act, the residents can access their own lab test results within 30 days of request _____. (p. 118)
    1. With their physician's permission
    2. With nursing personnel's permission
    3. If from a government lab
    4. Without going through the physician who ordered the test

37. The concept of lab-on-a-chip will _____. (p. 118)
    1. Speed up lab diagnoses in the nursing facility
    2. Eliminate the need for diagnoses
    3. Increase the cost of diagnoses
    4. Be done by the residents

38. Attempting to find the right person for each well-defined job is known as the management function of _____. (p. 3)
    1. Personnel work
    2. Interviewing
    3. Staffing
    4. The job search

39. The administrator who takes steps that ensure that the goals are accomplished and that each job is done as planned is successfully _____. (p. 5)
    1. Getting results
    2. Improving outputs
    3. Controlling quality
    4. Sensing organizational needs

40. The administrator's job is to ensure that the _____ employees do the tasks of the organization at an acceptable quality level. (*p. 4*)
    1. Best prepared
    2. Trained
    3. Appropriate
    4. Unmotivated

41. The administrator who conducts a national search for a director of nursing position and interviews 20 candidates from seven different surrounding states by phone is engaged in the managerial function of _____. (*p. 5*)
    1. Directing personnel development
    2. Staffing
    3. Broad personnel searches
    4. In-depth interviewing

42. In the end, it can be said that the administrator's responsibility to meet resident care needs and facility financial needs are _____. (*p. 6*)
    1. Clearly unequal
    2. A mismatch
    3. Both about equal
    4. Unclear

43. Superior performance depends on taking exceptional care of residents via superior service and _____. (*p. 6*)
    1. Constant attention to the bottom line
    2. Constant innovation
    3. Attention to detail
    4. A good attitude

44. Superior performance for a nursing facility comes through _____. (*p. 6*)
    1. Having all the beds full
    2. Achieving consistent profitability
    3. Innovation in ways to serve residents
    4. Efficient management of the budget

45. The superb nursing facility is superb by virtue of its _____. (*p. 6*)
    1. Success in attention to consistent profitability
    2. Success in serving the residents
    3. Reputation in the community as a friendly place
    4. Achieving superior ratings

46. Answering the phones and resident call bells with common courtesy and doing things that work are examples of _____. (*p. 6*)
    1. Good sense
    2. Uncommon perceptions
    3. An ability to be practical
    4. A blinding flash of the obvious

47. Giving every employee the space to innovate at least a little; listening to residents and acting on their ideas; and wandering around with residents, staff, and suppliers are examples of the difficult-to-achieve _____. (*p. 6*)
    1. Long-range goals
    2. Short-range goals
    3. Commonsense, obvious
    4. Typical facility approach

1.1.1 LEVELS OF MANAGEMENT

48. In a facility of 120 beds, the administrator _____ personally perform each of the management tasks. (*p. 7*)
    1. Need not
    2. Should
    3. Over a month will
    4. Over a year will

49. To ensure that all the management tasks are successfully accomplished, the administrator of a 120-bed facility will typically divide management into _____. (*p. 7*)
    1. Two layers
    2. Three layers
    3. Eight cooperating teams
    4. Four teams

50. A licensed person responsible for formulating and enforcing policies that will be applied to an entire facility is thought of as a/an _____. (*p. 7*)
    1. Upper level manager
    2. Senior administrator
    3. Board member
    4. Owner

51. The staff member responsible for reporting to upper-level management and at the same time interacting significantly with several lower-level managers is the _____. (*p. 7*)
    1. Director of finance
    2. Director of nursing
    3. Charge nurse
    4. Assistant to the administrator

52. The staff person for whom both upward and downward communication skills are the most necessary is the _____. (*p. 7*)
    1. Staff development coordinator
    2. Director of nursing
    3. Nursing supervisor
    4. Assistant administrator for personnel

53. When the director of nursing makes an effective policy decision without consulting the administrator that impacts all nursing personnel, the administrator should _____. (*p. 7*)
    1. Be pleased
    2. Nevertheless be somewhat concerned
    3. Counsel with the director of nursing about chain of command
    4. Begin the search for a new director of nursing

54. In the typical nursing facility, the decision-making process is _____ establishment of lower, middle, and upper levels of management. (*p. 8*)
    1. Noticeably more complicated than the simple
    2. Normally accomplished by the
    3. Successful if the ownership ensures effective
    4. Rendered relatively uncomplicated through

1.1.2 LINE–STAFF RELATIONSHIPS

55. Among the following positions, the _____ has no authority to make decisions for the facility. (*p. 8*)
    1. Director of nursing
    2. Supply room manager
    3. Assistant to the administrator
    4. Evening charge nurse

56. Decisions made by persons on the staff to whom the administrator has delegated line authority are, in the final analysis, regarded as decisions by _____. (*p. 8*)
    1. The owners
    2. The board of directors
    3. The administrator
    4. The department head holding such line authority

57. When a nurse practitioner, who is more highly qualified than the director of nursing, gives orders to nurses in the hallways, the director of nurses should feel _____. (*p. 9*)
    1. Reaffirmed
    2. Undermined
    3. That quality of care is being reinforced
    4. That a useful support system is functioning

58. In times of crisis, corporate representatives, who hold a staff or advisory relationship with their counterparts in the local facility, may expect that their advice as staff be _____. (*p. 9*)
    1. Regarded as strong recommendations
    2. Approached on a "take or leave it" basis
    3. Respected
    4. Acted on as carrying line authority

1.2 FORECASTING

59. As a generalization, it can be asserted that managerial success belongs to those who _____. (*p. 11*)
    1. Successfully prepare for the future
    2. Are reactive on every front
    3. Constantly take initiatives
    4. Conserve resources

60. Nursing home administrators should anticipate and successfully prepare for _____. (*p. 11*)
    1. Increased reimbursement
    2. New long-term care legislation
    3. Increased longevity
    4. Rapid change

61. The long-term care industry has entered a period in which _____ change(s) can be expected. (*p. 11*)
    1. Fewer
    2. More dramatic
    3. Rapid and far reaching
    4. A more controlled rate of

62. The ability to accurately predict the future implications for nursing facilities of new trends to which the present environment may offer small clues is the skill needed to successfully _____. (*p. 11*)
    1. Forecast
    2. Review
    3. Read the meaning of history
    4. Learn from the past

63. Historically, during the 1970s and early 1980s (until the introduction of the diagnosis-related group method [DRG] of reimbursement), nursing facility administrators made long-range projections during a period of _____. (*p. 11*)
    1. Unlimited change
    2. Intense social scrutiny of reimbursement mechanisms
    3. Relative stability in the health care field
    4. Rapid social change

64. The rate of change in the health care field is believed to be _____. (*p. 12*)
1. Slowing down
2. Coming under control
3. Increasing exponentially
4. Retrenching

65. Researchers have predicted that every 10 years _____ of all current knowledge and accepted practices in the health care and other industries will be _____. (*p. 12*)
1. One fourth/obsolete
2. One half/obsolete
3. Three fourths/still usable
4. Four fifths/still usable

66. It is conceivable that the core business of the nursing home in this decade will _____ the core business of the nursing home of the next decade. (*p. 12*)
1. Be entirely different from
2. Remain relatively stable and closely resemble
3. Undergo change at a slower pace than
4. Be remarkably similar to

67. One should expect that over the next few decades the rules governing the nursing home will be _____. (*p. 12*)
1. Relatively stable
2. New, never experienced before
3. Even more formalized by Congressional legislation
4. Enforced less due to decreased personnel available to state and federal agencies

68. Nursing homes that stick to conventional formulas for success are/will _____. (*p. 12*)
1. Be more likely to survive
2. Miss new markets and be in a backwash
3. Be more likely to produce a steady profit
4. Survive while those introducing constant change will lose needed focus

69. In the text it is argued that, for the first time in human history, the capacity exists to provide _____. (*p. 12*)
1. Complete health care for all citizens
2. A high level of health care for all citizens
3. More health care than any nation can afford
4. Affordable health care for all

70. The roles possible for hospitals, nursing homes, home health agencies, and managed care organizations are _____. (*p. 12*)
1. Predictable and, likely, manageable
2. Sorting themselves out
3. Being more and more successfully managed by government
4. Endless and will remain up for grabs

71. The staff in nursing facilities, over the next two decades, will likely _____. (*p. 12*)
    1. Experience culture shock
    2. Be reduced in staff/patient ratios
    3. Become accustomed to a predictable core business
    4. Remain committed to the facility, lowering turnover

1.3 PLANNING

1.3.1 WHY PLAN?

72. Plans can be said to be statements of the _____. (*p. 13*)
    1. Hopes of the administrator
    2. Hopes of the ownership
    3. Prediction of the next steps needed
    4. Organizational goals of the facility

73. In order to survive, each facility must _____. (*p. 13*)
    1. Deal with the outside world
    2. Have immeasurably more income than expenses
    3. Know what the future will bring years in advance
    4. Write enough policies to cover all contingencies

74. A major advantage associated with carefully developed plans is making it possible to _____. (*p. 13*)
    1. Control the future
    2. Not repeat past mistakes
    3. Compare what happens to what was predicted
    4. Compare what happens to past experiences

75. When external conditions change, plans _____. (*p. 13*)
    1. Should remain in place
    2. Can be altered to meet the changed conditions
    3. Should be monitored, but not radically altered
    4. Are of decreased value

76. Each facility's strategic plan must be endorsed by _____. (*p. 14*)
    1. The governing body
    2. The local health authority
    3. The state health department
    4. The federal or state surveyors

77. The average number of prescriptions for persons in the United States aged 65 years and older is six. In nursing facilities, it is _____. (*p. 14*)
    1. Lower
    2. About the same
    3. Often double that number
    4. Fewer due to closer medical monitoring

78. The observation about the idea that "if it ain't broke, don't fix it" is _____. (*p. 14*)
    1. That this is functionally valuable conventional wisdom
    2. That if it ain't broke today, it will be tomorrow
    3. That too few managers understand this good advice
    4. That this is a solid insight one can depend upon

79. The approach to planning known as SWOT refers to focusing on _____. (*p. 48*)
    1. Strengths, weaknesses, occupancy level, and threats
    2. Strategies, weaknesses, opportunities, and threats
    3. Strengths, weaknesses, opportunities, and threats
    4. Statistics, work options, opportunities, and trends

1.3.2 STEPS IN PLANNING

80. When considering building a new facility, necessary approvals by government agencies, such as zoning requirements, building codes, certificate of need, is/are _____. (*p. 15*)
    1. Routinely issued to applicants
    2. Sometimes difficult or impossible to obtain
    3. Available to all applicants
    4. Reserved for certain applicants

81. In general, government purposes and the facility goal of providing high-quality care are _____. (*p. 15*)
    1. Diverging in recent years
    2. The same
    3. Different
    4. Difficult to assess meaningfully

82. Looking at competitors' expansion plans, occupancy levels, and local hospital plans when considering building a nursing facility is known as conducting a _____. (*p. 16*)
    1. Needs assessment
    2. Review
    3. Constructive analysis
    4. Construction review

83. When planning a new nursing facility, the goal of being in operation within 4 months is best described as a/an _____. (*p. 17*)
    1. Unrealistic goal
    2. Long-range objective
    3. Short-range objective
    4. Realistic goal

84. As a general rule, the planning process moves from _____. (*p. 17*)
    1. Goal to goal
    2. Unrealistic to realistic
    3. General to specific
    4. Vague to sharp

85. One view of the planning process includes the observation that _____. (*p. 17*)
    1. The future will change our plans
    2. Keeping to a carefully thought-out plan is essential
    3. Planning produces a reasonable degree of certainty
    4. Plans, once in place, keep us on track toward our goal

86. Nursing home administrators who expect the unexpected and thrive on it _____. (*p. 17*)
    1. Exhibit an unnecessary anxiety about the future
    2. Are too pessimistic
    3. Will last in the profession
    4. Will not make enough plans

87. Facilities that embrace each new technology as it becomes available are known as _____. (*p. 18*)
    1. Correct
    2. Improvement oriented
    3. Early adapters
    4. The winners

88. The area offering the richest opportunities for innovation is _____. (*p. 17*)
    1. Nursing
    2. Financing
    3. The unexpected
    4. New trends

89. When one accepts the idea that change is a permanent part of life _____. (*p. 18*)
    1. Life becomes more uncontrollable
    2. Life becomes less comfortable
    3. Uncertainty proliferates
    4. One can take advantage of new opportunities

90. One must assume that other nursing home administrators in the community
_____. (*p. 17*)
1. Have found the best ways to "climb the mountain"
2. Are excellent marketers
3. May fail, if you fail
4. Are "searching for new ways to climb the mountain"

1.4 ORGANIZING

91. In the process of organizing the work of a facility, it is of real importance to
ensure that _____. (*p. 19*)
1. Workers are satisfied
2. Any union preferences are met
3. There is no duplication of work
4. Sufficient managers are appointed

92. Organizing is the first step in implementation of a/an _____. (*p. 19*)
1. Challenge to the workers
2. Plan
3. Organizational chart
4. Organizational reorganization

93. What the worker does, how the worker does it, what aids are necessary, what is
accomplished, and what skills are needed are parts of a _____. (*p. 19*)
1. Job family
2. Job review
3. Needs assessment
4. Job analysis

94. It can be argued that all nursing facility administrators organize their facility
according to _____. (*p. 19*)
1. Local requirements
2. The owners' needs·
3. Some theory of organization
4. The same theory of organization

95. Viewing organizations as systems has the advantage of offering the manager a
framework for visualizing the _____ of the organization. (*p. 19*)
1. Inputs
2. Outputs
3. Internal and external environment
4. Restraints

96. An organized or complex whole, an assembling or combining of things or parts forming a complex or single whole, best describes the _____. (*p. 19*)
    1. Systems concept
    2. Organizational theory concept
    3. Complexity concept
    4. Organizational chart concept

97. A primary advantage of systems theory is that it serves as a tool for making sense of the world by making clearer _____. (*p. 20*)
    1. How people interact
    2. Interrelationships within and outside the organization
    3. Interrelationships among the staff
    4. Interactions between staff and residents and their responsible parties

98. If the outputs of the organization do not meet the administrator's expectation he takes _____ actions to bring the outputs into line with those planned. (*p. 21*)
    1. Results-oriented
    2. Quick
    3. Effective
    4. Control

99. In essence, what nursing facilities do is use money to hire staff and provide materials needed to _____. (*p. 21*)
    1. Give patient care
    2. Show profitability
    3. Achieve conformity to regulations
    4. Meet owner requirements

100. The patient care that is given by the facility (i.e., the output) _____. (*p. 22*)
    1. Is usually good
    2. Can range from good to unacceptable
    3. Achieved cures for the residents
    4. Meets federal and state requirements

101. Asking if the work accomplished by the facility is up to expected standards and, if not, taking corrective actions is the act of _____. (*p. 23*)
    1. Taking charge
    2. Reviewing results
    3. Controlling quality
    4. Control of the inputs

102. The administrator uses _____ as the guidelines to compare the output with the expected results. (*p. 23*)
    1. The facility's policies and plans of action
    2. Goals
    3. Stated objectives
    4. External judgments

103. Allocating resources is the process of dividing resources among the various _____ of those resources. (*p. 21*)
    1. Claimants
    2. Current uses
    3. Traditional uses
    4. Competing possible uses

104. Optimizing resources is allocating resources with the result that _____ use is achieved. (*p. 21*)
    1. The fullest
    2. Most wanted
    3. Most effective possible
    4. Ever improving

105. Suppliers, bank creditors, visiting regulators, and advocacy groups can be thought of as _____ who evaluate the facility. (*p. 22*)
    1. Beneficiaries
    2. Potential regulators
    3. Clients
    4. Stakeholders

106. The most direct and immediate stakeholders within the facility are the _____. (*p. 22*)
    1. Family and personal representatives
    2. Immediate relatives
    3. Care recipients
    4. New hires

107. The passage of the Nursing Home Reform Act can be viewed as a form of _____ the nursing home industry. (*pp. 23–24*)
    1. Oppressive measure imposed on
    2. Object-oriented programming goals of
    3. External feedback of
    4. Internal feedback of

108. The external environment of the nursing facility consists of _____. (*p. 25*)
    1. Opportunities
    2. Initiatives available
    3. Constraints
    4. Opportunities and constraints

109. If something relates meaningfully to a nursing facility, but is something over which the facility has no control, for example, enforcement of the federal certification requirements, it can be said to be _____. (*p. 25*)
    1. Outside the facility's environment
    2. A constriction to the facility being successful
    3. A constraint in the external environment
    4. An opportunity

110. Increasing availability of managed care contracts, new niches, and increasing numbers of elderly needing care can be considered to be _____. (*p. 25*)
    1. Constraints
    2. Changes
    3. Opportunities
    4. Additional requirements

111. Systems analysis is most/equally useful to _____. (*p. 26*)
    1. The administrator
    2. The director of nursing
    3. The head of housekeeping
    4. The administrator, director of nursing, and head of housekeeping

112. Typically, the output of the nursing home as a system becomes the input for _____. (*p. 26*)
    1. Psychiatric hospitals
    2. Managed care organizations
    3. Health maintenance organizations
    4. The hospital or the resident's home

113. A nursing home and similar organizations can grow _____. (*p. 27*)
    1. Within a limited time span
    2. Until negative entropy applies
    3. Until resources run low
    4. Without any time limit

114. The entropy process is considered a universal law of nature that all organisms _____. (*p. 27*)
    1. Can grow indefinitely
    2. Move toward death
    3. Can expand
    4. Can expand as long as more inputs are available

115. As a general characteristic of organizations, it has been argued that, in general, organizations seek to _____. (*p. 28*)
    1. Grow
    2. Maintain their current size
    3. Shrink as needed
    4. Be flexible in adapting to change

116. Once in place, organizations become creatures of habit and develop a tendency to _____ change. (*p. 28*)
    1. Embrace
    2. Resist
    3. Build on
    4. Create

117. The most predictable response of a nursing facility experiencing a "disruptive employee" is to _____. (*p. 28*)
    1. Hold an inservice
    2. Counsel with the employee
    3. Let the employee go
    4. Contact the Equal Employment Opportunities Commission (EEOC) and ask for action

118. When a nursing facility chain goes from being the leader to being behind the pack, this can likely be attributed to _____. (*p. 29*)
    1. Bullheadedness of top management
    2. Overconfidence
    3. Lack of enthusiasm
    4. A deep reservoir of outmoded attitudes and policies

119. The training received in nursing school, medical school, and physical therapy school tends to _____. (*p. 29*)
    1. Create resistance to change
    2. Encourage innovation
    3. Open graduates to change
    4. Focus on niches

120. The real purpose of systems thinking is to _____. (*p. 29*)
    1. Empower people to introduce organizational change
    2. Ensure that the current adjustments remain
    3. Tutor employees in how the organization is arranged
    4. Achieve conformity to the organizational chart

1.5 STAFFING

121. The movement of American medicine from 80% general practitioners in 1870 to 20% general practitioners in the 2000s is an illustration of the tendency of organizations to _____. (*p. 29*)
    1. Grow increasingly complex
    2. Embrace change
    3. Reverse their ratios
    4. Achieve independence

1.6 DIRECTING

122. Directing is the process of communicating to employees what is to be done by each of them and _____. (*p. 31*)
    1. Enforcing the rules
    2. Rewriting the rules
    3. Helping them to accomplish it
    4. Providing active training courses

1.6.1 POLICY MAKING

123. It is _____ to make policies that direct the activities of employees everywhere in the facility 24 hours a day. (*p. 32*)
1. Impossible
2. Improbable
3. Possible
4. Undesirable

124. It is neither possible nor desirable to establish policies for _____. (*p. 33*)
1. All nursing assistants
2. The admissions coordinator
3. Every conceivable situation
4. Situations with some variability

125. The specific spelling out, step by step, of the intended implementation of a policy is known as a _____. (*p. 33*)
1. Set of controls
2. Detailing of policy
3. Set of procedures
4. Set of limits

126. A detailed plan of actions expected of each employee upon hearing the fire alarm is known as _____. (*p. 33*)
1. A clearly developed policy
2. A set of procedures
3. Management expectations
4. Detailed instructions

127. Normally, the _____ for the facility sets the mission and goals. (*p. 32*)
1. Family council
2. Executive committee
3. Governing body
4. Ombudsmen

128. Normally, the facility's role in implementing a facility's mission is to _____. (*p. 32*)
1. Originate ideas
2. Write and implement more specific policies and procedures
3. Edit as needed and implement
4. Combine owners' and residents' ideas

1.6.2 MAKING A DECISION

129. The internal process by which managers make decisions is _____. (*p. 38*)
    1. Well understood
    2. A subject of little interest
    3. Entirely subjective
    4. Imprecise, not well understood

130. It is the administrator's job to ensure that all employees make the right decisions for the facility _____. (*p. 38*)
    1. In every case
    2. With a minimum of worry
    3. Quickly
    4. As often as possible

131. Ethical practices throughout the facility are the _____responsibility. (*p. 39*)
    1. Owner's
    2. Stakeholder's
    3. Administrator's
    4. Director of nursing's

1.6.3 LEADING

132. Organizations that thrive over an extended period of time depend on having _____. (*p. 39*)
    1. Large profit margins
    2. Charismatic leadership
    3. Consistent leadership
    4. Effective leaders

133. Compared to defining the concept *deciding,* defining the concept *leading* is _____. (*p. 39*)
    1. Less difficult
    2. More difficult
    3. Much less difficult
    4. Researched and understood

134. The concept that history is *made* or measurably influenced by individuals who become leaders is known as _____. (*p. 39*)
    1. Leadership by men
    2. Leadership by innovators
    3. The great leadership theory of history
    4. Man the maker theory

135. Democratic, authoritarian, and laissez-faire are _____. (*p. 40*)
1. Types of leadership styles
2. Outmoded models for today's leaders
3. Discounted today
4. Types of political positions

136. A supervising staff member whom the administrator might most want to provide leadership by walking around is the _____. (*p. 41*)
1. Receptionist
2. Charge nurse
3. Director of nursing
4. Director of housekeeping

137. A major information advantage to leadership by walking around is the opportunity to _____. (*p. 41*)
1. Check on staff
2. Do naive listening
3. Get out of the office
4. Check the floors

138. It is _____ to maintain the chain of command when an administrator practices leadership by walking around. (*p. 41*)
1. Especially difficult
2. Especially easy
3. Entirely feasible
4. Impossible

139. An effective administrator does not overrule middle-level managers unless _____. (*p. 41*)
1. He or she personally disagrees
2. Harm could result
3. Management has specifically addressed that situation
4. Rules are not being fully observed

140. The administrator's work begins once the board has set forth the _____ of the organization. (*p. 40, 60*)
1. Full rules
2. Day-to-day rules and regulations
3. Mission statement
4. Procedures to be followed

141. The best time for the administrator to introduce change in the facility is when _____. (*p. 42*)
1. Everyone is ready for it
2. It is clear to all that the situation demands it
3. It will improve the bottom line
4. He or she does not have to

142. The better administrator is the one who _____. (*p. 42*)
1. Spends most hours in the facility wings
2. Is in his or her office constantly exploring ways to lead
3. Reviews reports as the primary information channel about the facility
4. Prepares for certification and the state to come in

143. For every successful decision the administrator makes _____. (*p. 42*)
1. The administrator is praised
2. Recognition comes from those affected
3. He or she may experience two or three wipeouts
4. Ownership is grateful

144. One thing the successful administrator remembers about the environment is that it _____. (*p. 42*)
1. Remains beyond control
2. Can be harnessed
3. Can be brought under control
4. Can be static

145. One reason for the administrator not to give all attention to the most immediate opportunity is that _____. (*p. 42*)
1. Corporate is unlikely to approve
2. Change costs too much energy
3. Better opportunities may also exist
4. It may not be what it seems

146. The best time to begin a move toward introducing a change into a facility is when _____. (*p. 42*)
1. Change is still on the horizon
2. Change is imminent
3. The climate is right
4. The staff are receptive

147. In the views of some contemporary corporate managers, change should be viewed more as a/an _____. (*p. 42*)
1. Continuous process, not an event
2. Process with some consistency
3. Predictable process that can be managed
4. Opportunity to consolidate past gains

148. Being knowledgeable about the field and having competence and experience will take today's administrator to _____. (*p. 43*)
1. Excellence
2. A good level
3. The highest level
4. Charismatic leadership

149. When nursing facility administrators have "that particular thing" in their blood they have a fire in the heart for _____. (*p. 43*)
    1. Continuous quality improvement
    2. Continuously improving the quality of daily life of each resident
    3. A successful career
    4. Being totally professional

150. Manager-centered leadership retains a _____ degree of control and uses _____ extensively. (*p. 44*)
    1. Low/authority
    2. Medium/authority
    3. High/authority
    4. High/charisma

151. Permitting subordinates to make the decision and function within the limits defined by the manager is closest to a _____ style of management. (*p. 44*)
    1. Laissez-faire
    2. Democratic
    3. Authoritarian
    4. Charismatic

152. When deciding what style of management to employ in a given situation, administrators should consider factors within themselves, factors in the employees, and factors in the _____. (*p. 45*)
    1. Organization
    2. External environment
    3. Five-year plan
    4. One-year plan

153. A manager who is responsible for the development of more specific policies that interpret administration's policies for the employees one supervises is closest to _____ managing. (*p. 45*)
    1. Upper-level
    2. Middle-level
    3. Lower-level
    4. Integrated

154. The charge nurse responsible for applying policies provided by the director of nursing services is functioning most closely at the _____ level of management. (*p. 45*)
    1. Upper
    2. Middle
    3. Lower
    4. Integrated

155. Origination, change, creation, and elimination of structure are the responsibility of _____ management. (*p. 46*)
    1. Upper-level
    2. Middle-level
    3. Lower-level
    4. Functional

156. Operational use of existing structure is the responsibility of _____ management. (*p. 46*)
    1. Upper-level
    2. Middle-level
    3. Lower-level
    4. Functional

157. Successful leaders need to be keenly aware of relevant forces in the situation, to understand themselves, and also _____ vis-à-vis the situation. (*p. 47*)
    1. Be calm and purposeful
    2. Interpret successfully
    3. Have insight
    4. Be able to behave appropriately

158. The acts of the _____ leader are typically unexamined. (*p. 49*)
    1. Accepted
    2. Venerated
    3. Charismatic
    4. Fully established

159. A valuable goal for each administrator is to deliver short-term results while securing _____. (*p. 48*)
    1. New friends
    2. High-level support
    3. Long-term viability
    4. Medium-term goals

1.6.4 POWER AND AUTHORITY

160. When one is able to motivate someone to do something he or she would not otherwise do, one is said to be wielding _____. (*p. 51*)
    1. Undue influence
    2. Self-control
    3. Power
    4. Excessive influence

161. In the American culture power is a/an _____. (*p. 51*)
    1. Relatively well-understood concept
    2. Accepted tradition for all members of society
    3. Complex concept
    4. Simple set of beliefs

162. The administrator's ability to award or withhold a year-end bonus represents _____ power held by the administrator. (*p. 52*)
    1. Punishment
    2. Overarching
    3. Financial
    4. Reward

163. Fear that the administrator may write a negative report and place it in one's personnel file represents the administrator's _____ power. (*p. 52*)
    1. Expert
    2. Personnel
    3. Controlling
    4. Punishment

164. Employees identifying and admiring the administrator yield _____ power to the administrator. (*p. 52*)
    1. Expert
    2. Exceptional
    3. Additional
    4. Referent

165. Two types of power available to all staff members are _____. (*p. 52*)
    1. Legitimate and reward
    2. Punishment and reward
    3. Referent and reward
    4. Expert and referent

166. As a general rule, it is better if an administrator can possess and exercise _____ power. (*p. 52*)
    1. Expert and referent
    2. Charismatic and punishment
    3. Expert and punishment
    4. Legitimate and punishment

167. The presence of numerous professions such as the medical, nursing, dental, and pharmaceutical professions in the facility tend to _____ the administrator's power. (*p. 53*)
    1. Constrain
    2. Increase
    3. Augment
    4. Supplement

1.6.5 COMMUNICATION SKILLS

168. Communication is the exchange of information and the transmission of _____.
(*p. 54*)
1. Meaning
2. Memos of documentation
3. Faxes
4. Internet messages

169. The administrator initiates a communication and it is transmitted from its source to its destination. Communication has _____. (*p. 55*)
1. Not yet taken place
2. Been accomplished
3. Been reviewed
4. Been retrieved

170. Listening with intensity, acceptance, empathy, and a willingness to assume responsibility for understanding the speaker's complete message is sometimes called _____. (*p. 55*)
1. Passive listening
2. Attentive listening
3. Active listening
4. Paying full attention

171. Two systems of communication usually exist side by side in an organization and are known as _____. (*p. 55*)
1. Active and inactive
2. Upward and lateral
3. First layer and second layer
4. Formal and informal

172. Two nurses chatting while on break in the nurse's lounge about a patient's status is _____ communication. (*p. 55*)
1. Upward
2. Downward
3. Horizontal
4. Peer

173. Two nurses chatting about the most recent events in the administrator's office while on break in the nurses' lounge are engaged in _____ communication. (*p. 55*)
1. Formal
2. Informal
3. Casual
4. Gossip-type

174. It can be reasonably argued that every communication is likely to have _____.
(*p. 55*)
1. Intended impact
2. Unintended consequences
3. Serendipitous results
4. Multiple levels of meaning

175. The informal communication process most closely resembles _____. (*p. 55*)
1. The consultant pharmacist reporting findings to the director of nursing
2. The nurse assistant chatting with a resident while making the bed
3. The administrator calling a report in to corporate
4. The charge nurse reporting to the nurse supervisor

176. The director of nursing giving instructions to the nurse supervisor is considered _____. (*p. 55*)
1. Upward communication
2. Downward communication
3. Flawed communication
4. To be done twice each shift

177. The nurse assistant reporting to the nurse supervisor about an incident in a patient room is an example of _____ communication. (*p. 55*)
1. Upward
2. Downward
3. Optional
4. Well-organized

178. The closer one gets to the organization center of control, the administrator's office, for example, the _____. (*p. 55*)
1. More pronounced the emphasis is on the exchange of information
2. Less important constant information exchange becomes
3. Less necessary written reports become
4. More comfortably the administrator can operate

179. The nurse assistant, preoccupied and angry over unsettled matters at home, interprets the comments by the nurse as hostile comments. This illustrates a barrier to communication known as _____. (*p. 56*)
1. Differences in knowledge level
2. Subgroup allegiance
3. Status distance
4. Agenda carrying

180. The charge nurse who remembers the words of praise from the director of nursing but ignores the criticisms also received from the director of nursing illustrates a barrier to communication known as _____. (*p. 56*)
    1. Selective hearing
    2. Subgroup allegiance
    3. Status distance
    4. Agenda carrying

181. A nurse assistant realizes that her fellow nurse assistant is sleeping much of the night shift, but decides not to report her. This illustrates _____. (*p. 56*)
    1. Differences in knowledge level
    2. Subgroup allegiance
    3. Status distance
    4. The filter effect

182. The nurse's aide realized that the patient's condition should be pointed out to the attending physician who had just popped into the patient's room, but hesitated to approach the physician. This illustrates the effects of _____. (*p. 57*)
    1. Differences in knowledge level
    2. Subgroup allegiance
    3. Status distance
    4. The filter effect

183. The medication nurse thought she understood what the pharmacist had just said about the side effects of a medication, but found the technical jargon used by the pharmacist to be intimidating. This illustrates _____. (*p. 57*)
    1. Differences in knowledge level
    2. The language barrier
    3. Status distance
    4. The filter effect

184. The charge nurse decided not to write up an incident on her shift because four incidents had already been written up that week on her shift. This illustrates _____. (*p. 57*)
    1. Differences in knowledge level
    2. Subgroup allegiance
    3. Self-protection
    4. The filter effect

185. The new 30-page-long policy on universal precautions contained so many new requirements that staff soon began to revert to their time-tested approaches in conducting patient care. This illustrates _____. (*p. 57*)
    1. Differences in knowledge level
    2. Information overload
    3. Status distance
    4. The filter effect

1.6.6 ORGANIZATIONAL NORMS AND VALUES: CODE OF ETHICS AND STANDARDS OF PRACTICE

186. Under Tag F241 the government defines dignity as caring for residents in a manner that maintains full recognition of the resident's _____. (*p. 59*)
    1. Individuality
    2. Personal tastes
    3. Past types of activities
    4. Reasonable expectations

187. Dignity has been interpreted by states' examiners _____. (*p. 60*)
    1. With wide variations
    2. Fairly consistently
    3. Differently depending on the section of the country
    4. With excellent consistency

188. Standardized patterns of required behaviors developed by the facility to enable staff to accomplish necessary work defines a _____. (*p. 59*)
    1. Norm
    2. Set of values
    3. Specific patterns
    4. Role

189. Since about the year 2000, the percentage of nursing facilities in the United States given deficiencies in quality of life, dignity _____. (*p. 59*)
    1. Held steady
    2. Went consistently up
    3. Varied widely by state and over time
    4. Went lower as facilities improved care

190. Treating all residents with respect is best described as a _____. (*p. 59*)
    1. Role
    2. Norm
    3. Value
    4. Commitment

191. A statement broadly defining the purposes and values held by a facility is a _____. (*p. 60*)
    1. Statement of intent
    2. Set of aspirations
    3. Long-term goal
    4. Mission statement

192. When the administrator concentrates on getting paperwork done, meeting regulations, and saving money, the staff _____. (*p. 60*)
    1. Are freed to give more attention to good patient care
    2. Do the same
    3. Feel the facility is being successfully managed
    4. Give better quality care

193. The area in which it is especially important for the administrator to implement a "no excuses" approach is _____. (*p. 60*)
    1. In preventive maintenance
    2. In projecting capital needs
    3. Patient care
    4. Staff attitudes

194. It is easier for staff to buy into and be motivated by a _____. (*p. 61*)
    1. Day-to-day set of achievements to be reached
    2. Well-organized administrator
    3. Well-motivated administrator
    4. Dream or vision

195. If a facility administrator can communicate a vision or dream _____. (*p. 61*)
    1. Goals are less necessary
    2. Goals can be more easily set and achieved
    3. Employee tenure will be maintained
    4. Employees will stop focusing on pay rates

196. Each state legislature publishes standards of practice and sets the _____ behavior expectations for nursing home administrators. (*p. 60*)
    1. Legalistic
    2. Most forceful
    3. Ethical
    4. Fully agreed upon

197. Corporate-generated goals or mission statements generally _____. (*p. 61*)
    1. Motivate local facility workers
    2. Enervate
    3. Innovate
    4. Have difficulty motivating local facility workers

198. Organizations need the leadership of the administrator because, in the final analysis, _____. (*p. 61*)
    1. The administrator knows what is best
    2. People need to be led
    3. Someone has to be in charge
    4. All organizational designs are imperfect

199. The actual behavior and functioning of an organization such as a nursing facility _____. (*p. 61*)
1. Closely resemble the plan
2. Are an implementation of the plan
3. Are relatively easily achieved
4. Are infinitely more complex and incomplete than the plan

1.6.7 RELATED CONCEPTS

200. The concept of delegation is permitting decisions to be made _____. (*p. 63*)
1. With full information
2. By the well-qualified nurse
3. At the lowest level possible
4. At the middle level of management

201. How people relate to each other in the organization and the overall style or feel of an organization are referred to as _____. (*p. 62*)
1. Corporate meaning
2. The value system
3. The corporate culture
4. The personnel handbook mission statement

202. The concept of unity of command emphasizes the importance of each person _____. (*p. 63*)
1. Feeling like he or she fits in
2. Remaining on the team
3. Having a meaningful role in the organization
4. Being accountable to one supervisor

203. When the board of directors gives equal authority to manage the facility to the medical director and the administrator, the board has ignored the _____ concept. (*p. 63*)
1. Short chain of command
2. Utility
3. Delegation
4. Unity of command

204. The principle that there should be as few levels of management between the chief administrator and the rank and file is the _____. (*p. 63*)
1. Short chain of command
2. Intervening levels
3. Effective middle levels of managers
4. Maximum use of managers

205. When the number of interpreters through whom information must be filtered before it reaches top management is minimized, the concept of _____ has been implemented. (*p. 63*)
  1. Balance
  2. Span of control
  3. Short chain of command
  4. Low profile

206. The administrator who pays attention to the size of the various departments, centralization and decentralization, span of control, and short chain of command is paying attention to _____. (*p. 64*)
  1. Being a good manager
  2. Being effective
  3. The concept of balance
  4. What is occurring in the facility

207. The administrator who begins with the nursing assistants' ideas then moves upward through the director of nursing's ideas and does so for each department is utilizing the concept of _____. (*p. 64*)
  1. Management information systems
  2. Lowest to highest
  3. Respect for the individual worker
  4. Management by objectives

208. In determining the need for information; sources of information; and the amount, form, and frequency of information, the administrator is considering his or her _____. (*p. 64*)
  1. Idea sources
  2. Ways of organizing the facility
  3. Management information system
  4. Record-keeping measures

209. The administrator tells the admissions director to drop the daily reporting and to report only on days census drops below 90%. The administrator is utilizing the _____ concept. (*p. 65*)
  1. Program Evaluation and Review Technique (PERT)/Critical Path Method (CPM)
  2. Delegation
  3. Management by objectives
  4. Management by exception

210. Mapping out time estimates for the completion of each step in renovating a wing is using _____. (*p. 65*)
  1. Program Evaluation and Review Technique (PERT)/Critical Path Method (CPM)
  2. Delegation
  3. Management by objectives
  4. Management by exception

211. The administrator in the chain who is achieving the best level of resident care, but not necessarily the lowest cost per patient day, can be said to be _____, although perhaps not the most efficient administrator. (*p. 65*)
   1. Most acceptable
   2. Effective
   3. Best motivated
   4. The best producer

212. Studies of top corporate administrators suggest that these persons feel that they can _____. (*p. 66*)
   1. Manage best in their industry
   2. Train anyone to become a top manager
   3. Be motivators for everyone in the organization
   4. Manage almost anything

213. The administrator who focuses on the time it takes for each housekeeper to clean an area and the time it takes for a nurse assistant to make a bed identifies with the _____. (*p. 66*)
   1. Necessity to conserve time
   2. Necessity to be effective
   3. Scientific management school
   4. Human relations school

214. Administrators who believe that human factors exercise the most powerful influences due to worker need to participate in social groups identify with the _____ school of management theory. (*p. 67*)
   1. Scientific
   2. Practical
   3. Theoretical
   4. Human relations

215. Security of residents' medical records is of special concern because it is covered under _____. (*p. 68*)
   1. Most state rules
   2. All state rules
   3. Health department rules
   4. HIPAA

216. Encoding data into unrecognizable streams of data while data are in transit is known as _____. (*p. 68*)
   1. A prudent business practice
   2. Good data management
   3. Information technology
   4. Cryptology

217. Web-based technologies to create interactive platforms through which individuals and communities share, create, and discuss ideas is known as _____. (*p. 69*)
   1. Information technology
   2. Social media
   3. Emerging tools
   4. Best practices

1.7 COMPARING AND CONTROLLING QUALITY

218. An administrator judging the extent of actual results of the facility's efforts to achieve the outcomes proposed in its plans is _____. (*p. 70*)
   1. Reviewing
   2. Judging
   3. Achievement oriented
   4. Comparing

219. The administrator who is successfully taking the steps necessary to adjust policies and plans of action to more satisfactorily achieve stated goals is engaged in _____. (*p. 70*)
   1. Active managing
   2. Controlling
   3. Implementing
   4. Conserving resources

220. Translating goals into clearly stated policies, identifying appropriate measures, and stating limits to deviation are some of the requirements for _____. (*pp. 70–71*)
   1. Improving management
   2. Effective control of quality
   3. Getting ahead of competitors
   4. Managing for results

221. Getting information in a useful form to staff at appropriate levels, stating policies of actions to be taken when limits are exceeded, and taking corrective actions are some of the requirements for _____. (*p. 71*)
   1. Improving management
   2. Effective control of quality
   3. Getting ahead of competitors
   4. Managing for results

222. Setting up a system for constant renewal of quality measures, finding control measures that are functional and valued by staff, and knowing the limitations of the scope and capabilities of a system are some of the requirements for _____. (p. 71)
    1. Improving management
    2. Effective control of quality
    3. Getting ahead of competitors
    4. Managing for results

1.7.2 DIAGNOSING/ORGANIZATIONAL QUALITY

223. Physicians diagnose and treat patient illnesses; administrators diagnose and treat _____ illnesses. (p. 72)
    1. Staff
    2. Corporate
    3. Organizational
    4. Epidemic

224. When an administrator studies and determines what is believed to be a problem adversely affecting the nursing facility, the administrator is engaged in a study of _____. (p. 72)
    1. Human nature
    2. What motivates employees
    3. Organizational pathology
    4. Organizational attitudes

225. Which of the following is not a federal quality measure? _____. (p. 72)
    1. Percent of staff having a good feeling about patients
    2. Percent of residents who need help with activities of daily living
    3. Percent of residents with urinary tract infections
    4. Percent of short-stay residents with pressure sores

226. Managers have always sought to achieve quality control in their organizations and _____. (p. 72)
    1. Clear successes have been attained across the board
    2. The need for such control is a subject of controversy
    3. This remains an elusive aspect of managing
    4. This is largely a thing of the past since the turn of the century

227. Ensuring that all the organizational arrangements believed to be needed are in place puts the emphasis on _____ as a quality measure. (p. 78)
    1. Structure
    2. Process
    3. Outcome
    4. Productivity

228. Focusing on the results of the effort made and the measurable impact on the patient given care places the emphasis on _____ as a quality measure. (*p. 79*)
    1. Structure
    2. Process
    3. Outcome
    4. Productivity

229. The federal focus on the idea that a resident's abilities in activities of daily living do not diminish unless circumstances indicate it is unavoidable places the focus on _____. (*p. 79*)
    1. Structure
    2. Process
    3. Outcome measures
    4. Productivity

230. Quality, argued Deming, comes from _____. (*p. 74*)
    1. Constant inspections
    2. A low rework rate
    3. Improvement in the process
    4. Unswerving attention

231. Deming observed that too often nurses and nurse's aides _____. (*p. 74*)
    1. Did not really care about doing a quality job
    2. Did not identify with the goals of the facility
    3. Learned their job from workers who were never trained properly
    4. Learned too much in nursing and nursing assistant training

232. The nurse supervisor's job, according to Deming, is to _____. (*p. 74*)
    1. Lead
    2. Train properly
    3. Set standards
    4. Require commitment

233. An atmosphere, according to Deming, in which employees feel secure enough to ask questions, take positions, and admit errors is free of _____. (*p. 74*)
    1. Serious mistakes
    2. Arguments
    3. Fear
    4. Refusal to work

234. The best source of slogans or work goals, in Deming's view, is _____. (*p. 74*)
    1. Corporate leadership
    2. The community
    3. The facility
    4. Each individual worker

235. Deming would _____ (of) setting the number of beds to be made each day or the number of rooms to be cleaned or floors scrubbed. (*pp. 74–75*)
1. Approve
2. Disapprove
3. Insist on
4. See as quite functional the

236. In Deming's view, workers are _____. (*p. 75*)
1. Eager to do a good job
2. In need of constant retraining
3. Uninterested in the overall goals of the business
4. Unmotivated for the most part

237. Evaluation by performance, merit rating, and annual review of performance, in Deming's view, _____. (*p. 75*)
1. Encourages workers
2. Allows workers to know where they stand
3. Is regarded by workers as fair and needed
4. Destroys teamwork and nurture rivalry

238. If the administrator tells the director of nursing to compare how the facility's nursing services are organized with what is considered the best organized nursing services in the area, the administrator is _____. (*p. 76*)
1. Comparing
2. Contrasting
3. Benchmarking
4. Trying to improve

239. A benchmarking effort _____ be justified by seeking out significantly better practices rather than solely focusing on best practices. (*p. 76*)
1. Can rarely
2. Can
3. Never is
4. Always can

240. When Deming warned not to simply copy others' efforts when benchmarking, he was advocating _____. (*p. 77*)
1. A new approach to benchmarking
2. Less benchmarking
3. Improved benchmarking
4. Adapting, rather than copying, benchmarked ideas

241. Total organizational involvement in improving all aspects of quality of service is the goal of _____. (*p. 77*)
1. Total quality management
2. New management
3. Spectrum management
4. Management by objective

242. The approach in total quality of management of placing responsibility with the workers who produce a service is sometimes known as _____. (*p. 77*)
    1. Source management
    2. Outsourcing
    3. Quality at the source
    4. Worker involvement

243. Employee empowerment in decision making, use of teams, and use of individual responsibility for services characterizes _____. (*p. 77*)
    1. Management by quality
    2. Resource maximization
    3. Total quality management
    4. Benchmarking

244. In the American Hospital Association's view, the goal of total quality management is to _____ customer expectations. (*p. 78*)
    1. Meet
    2. Anticipate
    3. Exceed
    4. Analyze

245. Visionary chief executive officers (CEOs) acting as coaches, commitment to customers, and trained teams characterize _____. (*p. 77*)
    1. Successful benchmarking
    2. The Deming analysis and recommendation
    3. Total quality management
    4. Management by objectives

246. Managing for quality consists of quality planning, quality control, and _____. (*pp. 80–81*)
    1. Knowing the difference
    2. Being able to see the difference
    3. Quality improvement
    4. Benchmarking

1.8 INNOVATING

247. Bringing new ideas into the way an organization accomplishes its purposes is the result of _____. (*p. 85*)
    1. Hard work
    2. Predicting the future
    3. Innovating
    4. Quality improvement

248. The role of innovator is _____. (*p. 85*)
1. Best assigned to the administrator
2. Available to all employees
3. A skill employees are able to develop
4. Best taught in inservices

249. One writer suggests that managers should _____ specific objectives that will guide the organization over an extended period of time. (*p. 85*)
1. Avoid trying to set out too
2. Encourage
3. Assign
4. Insist on

250. In the nursing facility, innovation is _____. (*p. 86*)
1. Seldom encountered
2. The prerogative of middle and upper management
3. Finding new solutions to creating quality of life for residents
4. An ever-elusive goal

251. Innovation can be expected _____. (*p. 86*)
1. From all levels in a nursing home chain
2. Primarily from upper-level management
3. Primarily from ownership
4. From middle-level well-trained staff who have the opportunity to update their skills

252. Google's Android and Apple's iOS have facilitated unprecedented development of _____. (*p. 87*)
1. Communication
2. Apps
3. Software
4. Future possibilities

253. In the nursing facility, the microphone on the smartphone can be used to quantify components of _____. (*p. 87*)
1. Liver function
2. Lung function
3. Endocrine presence or absence
4. Brain function

254. In the near future, ultrasound will be available to _____. (*p. 88*)
1. The local ER
2. The urgent care centers
3. The emergent care center
4. Nursing home nurses

255. Daughters and the government are increasingly likely to _____ timely diagnosis of changes in health conditions. (*p. 88*)
1. Force nursing facilities into
2. Preclude the progress of
3. Sue the facility for
4. Preclude

256. Due to new technologies, health care provided by nursing facilities will be increasingly _____. (*p. 88*)
1. Uni-level
2. Multilayered
3. Error prone
4. Totally comprehensive

257. A social graph of information such as demographics, location, family, likes, are part of the medical information of the future known as the _____. (*p. 88*)
1. Physiome
2. Atanome
3. Phenome
4. Exosome

258. The resident's individual anatomy, documenting the individual's heterogeneity is one's _____. (*p. 89*)
1. Protenome
2. Phenome
3. Anatome
4. Metabolome

259. All the environmental exposures the resident has experienced are described as the resident's _____. (*p. 89*)
1. Phenome
2. Exosome
3. Metabolome
4. Protenome

1.9 MARKETING THE LONG-TERM CARE FACILITY

1.9.1 THE TURN TO MARKETING

260. Like many hospitals, nursing homes are increasingly turning to _____ to maintain satisfactory income. (*p. 90*)
1. Corporate bonds
2. Filling a market niche
3. Stock offerings
4. Increasing the profit margins achieved

261. When a facility has achieved the premier status as the best caregiver in the community, experience suggests that it will likely _____. (*p. 91*)
    1. Retain that position over time
    2. Lull itself into complacency
    3. Make an even greater effort to retain its position
    4. Seek additional ways to maintain that position

262. In today's competitive market, good nursing facilities _____. (*p. 91*)
    1. Abound
    2. Are scarce
    3. Seldom are identifiable
    4. Have disappeared

263. The downside of being a good nursing facility is that it _____. (*p. 91*)
    1. Causes staff to stop trying
    2. Is difficult to maintain
    3. Is not recognized by the public
    4. Only puts you with the rest of the pack

1.9.2 THE "MARKETING" OF HEALTH CARE

264. Several years ago, the U.S. Supreme Court _____ self-imposed restrictions by health and other professionals against advertising services or prices that result in keeping the public ignorant or inhibiting free flow of information. (*p. 91*)
    1. Ruled as permissible
    2. Discouraged, but did not rule illegal
    3. Ruled illegal
    4. Permitted

265. Competition occurs when two or more organizations seek to serve _____ in an exchange process. (*p. 92*)
    1. Two or more groups
    2. Four or more groups
    3. Numerous individuals
    4. The same individual or group

266. The audit, market segmentation, choosing a market mix, implementing the plan, evaluation of results, and control are the steps in _____ . (*p. 92*)
    1. Managing by objectives
    2. Total quality management
    3. Marketing
    4. Good management

267. The marketing of the nursing facility is in a special context because of _____.
(*p. 93*)
1. Special laws covering nursing facility marketing
2. Public ambivalence toward the nursing facility
3. Special costs to the nursing facility not borne by other providers
4. Restrictive legislation governing nursing facility marketing practices

1.9.3 DEVELOPING A MARKETING STRATEGY

268. Selecting a target market or markets, choosing a competitive position, and developing an effective marketing mix to reach and serve the identified customers is _____. (*p. 94*)
1. Unnecessary for the typical nursing facility
2. Necessary only in states where no certificate of need exists
3. Developing a marketing strategy
4. Implementing good planning and directing

269. A marketing strategy includes _____. (*p. 94*)
1. Excessive sums of money
2. Hiring an outside firm
3. Hiring a marketing person
4. Selecting a target

270. The administrator asks a committee to engage in the process of identifying, collecting, and analyzing information about the external environment. In marketing terminology, the administrator is seeking a/an _____. (*p. 97*)
1. Environmental analysis
2. Audit
3. Segmented market
4. Multiple market

271. When the administrator decides to serve only longer-term residents, Medicare residents, and Alzheimer residents, in marketing terminology, the administrator has selected the _____. (*p. 98*)
1. Product mix
2. Targets
3. Goals
4. Opportunities

272. The steps of problem recognition, information search, alternative evaluation, purchase decision, and post-purchase evaluation are, in marketing texts, identified as the steps in _____. (*p. 99*)
1. Consumer decision making
2. Facility market segmentation decisions
3. Health care marketing practices
4. Government rule making

273. Factors such as general appearance of the facility, absence of odors, and the appearance of the patients may be those about which the decision maker may not be consciously aware while visiting a facility into which to place a relative. These are referred to as _____ factors. (*p. 100*)
1. Key
2. Special
3. Usual
4. Subliminal

274. Normally, one of the most effective marketing tools is _____. (*p. 100*)
1. Advertising
2. Staff recommendations
3. A tour through the facility
4. Hiring a consultant

275. Cognitive readiness, affective readiness, and behavioral readiness are _____. (*p. 100*)
1. A complex marketing theory
2. The steps in marketing
3. The goals of advertising
4. Often not cost-effective

276. Which staff should normally talk to the press? (*p. 101*)
1. The marketing person
2. The administrator
3. Only the owner
4. Any qualified and knowledgeable persons

NAB Domain: Human Resources

Understanding the Departments and Managing Human Resources

2.1 ORGANIZATION OF THE NURSING FACILITY AND ITS STAFF: EMERGENCE OF THE "MDS" COORDINATOR*

1. One practical reason the administrator must rely more and more on the expertise of department heads is _____. (*p. 108*)
   1. Requirements are too numerous for one person to remember
   2. Department heads are better trained
   3. Department heads come with more experience
   4. Department heads care more

2. One overarching consideration in deciding at what level, that is, the number of nursing hours per patient day, to staff the facility is _____. (*p. 108*)
   1. Ownership needs
   2. Medical complexity of care given
   3. Number of patients
   4. State and federal minimum staffing requirements

3. The one person most responsible for resident rights in the nursing facility is the _____. (*p. 111*)
   1. Administrator
   2. Direct caregiver
   3. Director of nursing
   4. Resident council president

4. Quality assessment and control, infection control, and physical plant health and safety are _____. (*p. 109*)
   1. New requirements
   2. Long-standing requirements
   3. Federally required committees
   4. Federally required committees and/or functions

---

*Answers can be found in *Nursing Home Administration*, Seventh Edition, on the page numbers in parentheses following each question.

5. Generally, the percentage of nursing facilities with deficiencies for resident rights in 2015 was _____. (*p. 111*)
    1. More than 15
    2. Unacceptable
    3. Less than 3
    4. Less than 15

6. In the typical nursing facility of 100 patients, the administrator normally has _____ reporting to him or her. (*p. 110*)
    1. Seventeen department heads
    2. Six middle-level managers
    3. Eight or nine department heads
    4. Three or four department heads

7. Larger facilities (200 or more patients) might consider the appointment of perhaps _____ middle-level managers to whom two or more department heads may report. (*p. 110*)
    1. Two
    2. Three
    3. Four
    4. Half a dozen

8. Activities such as ensuring quality of care for all residents, advocating for all residents, and developing and managing the budget are normally associated most closely with the _____. (*p. 110*)
    1. Business office
    2. Admissions team
    3. Nursing area
    4. Administrator's office

9. In 2015, U.S. nursing facilities achieved _____ compliance with physician services. (*p. 114*)
    1. 50%
    2. 60%
    3. 75%
    4. 98% or more

10. Activities such as empowering department heads, setting the tone, and settling territorial disputes are normally associated most closely with the _____. (*p. 111*)
    1. Business office
    2. Admissions team
    3. Nursing area
    4. Administrator's office

11. The rate of compliance with dental requirements in U.S. facilities in 2015 was
    _____. (p. 116)
    1. Less than 50%
    2. 80%
    3. 99%
    4. 100%

12. Federal, congressionally written requirements for the role(s) the medical direc-
    tor may/must play are _____. (p. 114)
    1. Brief and vague
    2. Detailed and extensive
    3. Constantly changing
    4. Becoming increasingly burdensome in recent years

13. When attending physicians fail to visit their patients on a timely basis, the med-
    ical director _____. (p. 113)
    1. Often substitutes and accomplishes the required physician services
    2. Never substitutes
    3. Must send federally required reminder notices
    4. Must provide mandatory counseling with these physicians

14. In most nursing facilities of 100 to 200 beds, there is _____ medical staff. (p. 114)
    1. Always an organized
    2. Usually no organized
    3. An open
    4. A closed

15. Pharmacy services in U.S. nursing facilities in 2015 were about 98% in compli-
    ance with the exception of _____. (p. 117)
    1. Procedures and storage
    2. Drug passes
    3. Record keeping
    4. Giving medications on a timely basis

16. One of the main advantages of a closed medical staff is that _____. (p. 114)
    1. One of the staff can be on call all the time
    2. Cost savings are realized
    3. Patients are more satisfied with the care given
    4. Patients like the broader choice available

17. Facility compliance with laboratory services requirements in 2015 was _____.
    (p. 119)
    1. Less than previous years
    2. The basis for closing several facilities
    3. About 75%
    4. Nearly 100%

18. Closed medical staffs are more likely in _____ facilities that serve a large _____ patient population. (*p. 114*)
    1. Smaller/Medicare
    2. Medium-sized/Medicare
    3. Larger/Medicare
    4. Larger/Medicaid

19. Dental care is often a neglected area of care in nursing facilities because dentists _____. (*p. 115*)
    1. Are typically reimbursed approximately half the office fee
    2. Are not interested in the geriatric population
    3. Feel less care is needed in the geriatric population
    4. Are not trained to care for older persons

20. Dental care is also often a neglected area of care in nursing facilities because dentists _____. (*p. 115*)
    1. Are often insecure about functioning outside their office with complex cases
    2. Are not eligible for Medicare reimbursement
    3. Are not eligible for Medicaid reimbursement
    4. Are nearly all overworked and have no time available

21. Total registered nurse (RN) and licensed practical nurse (LPN) hours per patient day in U.S. nursing facilities during 1993 to 2015 _____. (*p. 120*)
    1. Remained unchanged
    2. Rose perceptibly and then decreased slightly
    3. Decreased
    4. Reflected the nursing shortage

22. Successful solutions to oral care in the facility will likely be linked to _____. (*p. 115*)
    1. Training a local dentist
    2. Paying a rate higher than the office rate
    3. Retaining a dental director at perhaps $5.00 to $8.00 per patient per month
    4. Arranging for care through the local dental school

23. There is need in most nursing facilities for a _____ who will make rounds, see patients on a monthly basis, and train nursing staff to observe and meet patients' oral needs. (*p. 115*)
    1. Dental technician
    2. Dentist
    3. Dental assistant
    4. Dental hygienist

24. One practical solution to attaining a satisfactory level of oral care for nursing facility patients is to _____. (*p. 115*)
    1. Contract with several dentists for weekly visits
    2. Hire two or three dental hygienists
    3. Train oral care aides (a regularly employed nurse's aide)
    4. Seek Medicaid reimbursement for oral care given

25. A podiatrist is an important component of foot care in the nursing facility because _____. (*p. 116*)
    1. People like good care of their feet
    2. Residents walk a lot
    3. Diabetics need podiatrists for safe toenail clipping
    4. Medicaid requires it on a monthly basis

26. Ensuring all medications are available as ordered, that all reorders and stop orders are implemented, and reviewing each patient's medications monthly falls to the _____. (*p. 116*)
    1. Local pharmacy
    2. Pharmacists providing medications to the facility
    3. Director of nursing
    4. Consulting pharmacist

27. Observing medication passes and recording and reporting drug error rates falls to the _____. (*p. 117*)
    1. Director of nursing
    2. Consulting pharmacist
    3. Administrator's office
    4. Medical director

28. A facility of 120 patients with eight new admissions per month might _____ physical therapy services. (*p. 117*)
    1. Contract for
    2. Provide in-house
    3. Routinely send residents out for
    4. Not offer

29. A facility of 120 patients with 30 to 40 new admissions each month would likely _____ physical therapy services. (*p. 117*)
    1. Offer in-house
    2. Contract for a few hours per week any
    3. Not offer
    4. Routinely send residents out for

30. One way some facilities have bridged the gap between formal physical therapy given and the "habilitative" care given daily by the nursing staff is to _____. (p. 118)
    1. Place a physical therapist on staff
    2. Use an occupational therapist as well
    3. Train all nurses in physical therapy
    4. Establish a restorative nursing program led by a nurse

31. Increasingly, facilities needing x-rays are _____. (p. 118)
    1. Calling 911
    2. Using local buses for the handicapped
    3. Using mobile x-ray services
    4. Installing their own x-ray department with staff

32. In the nursing facility, implanted ports, midline catheters, central-line catheters, and epidural lines are part of _____. (p. 122)
    1. Routine nursing
    2. Intensive care unit nursing
    3. Subacute care
    4. New wave health care

33. For nursing to achieve its tasks _____. (p. 126)
    1. Nearly every department must cooperate
    2. Well-trained staff are desirable
    3. In-services must be routine
    4. Nurses must care deeply

34. Keeping medical records must be assigned to _____. (p. 128)
    1. A part-time employee
    2. A well-trained employee
    3. A medical records specialist
    4. A full-time employee

35. The major difference between the challenge faced by the nursing home dietary director compared with the hospital dietary director is _____. (p. 129)
    1. Fewer patients to feed
    2. Fewer staff
    3. Diets over an extended period of time
    4. Patient preferences

36. During the years 1993 to 2006, the major area in dietary services that needed improvement in the view of the inspectors was _____. (p. 132)
    1. Taste of the food
    2. Sanitary conditions
    3. Presentation of food
    4. Feeding styles

37. A particular patient care-related concern the administrator should address when evaluating the social worker's and activities director's work is _____. (*p. 136*)
    1. Whether they are well trained
    2. Whether they like their jobs
    3. Whether less responsive patients are receiving attention
    4. How well they interact with other staff

38. Deficiencies for housekeeping appear to be _____. (*p. 143*)
    1. Varying over time
    2. Going up
    3. Degrading
    4. Fully acceptable

2.2 IDENTIFYING THE HUMAN RESOURCES FUNCTIONS

39. The personnel for whom the personnel director has line responsibility is _____. (*p. 147*)
    1. All staff
    2. Staff outside of the nursing area
    3. Personnel department staff
    4. New hires still in the 90-day initial employment period

40. In practice, most of the actual hiring in nursing facilities is done by the _____. (*p. 147*)
    1. Director of personnel
    2. Director of nursing
    3. Administrator
    4. Department managers

41. In the typical facility of 100 patients there is(are) _____ full-time personnel director(s). (*p. 147*)
    1. One
    2. Two
    3. No
    4. A professionally trained

2.3 PLANNING EMPLOYMENT NEEDS: WRITING JOB DESCRIPTIONS

42. The process of defining a job in terms of tasks or behaviors required and specifying the qualifications is performing a _____. (*p. 149*)
    1. Job specification
    2. Job description
    3. Job analysis
    4. Job evaluation

43. Information about the job that results in a statement of the job to be done including a list of duties, title, and qualifications is a job _____. (*p. 149*)
    1. Specification
    2. Description
    3. Analysis
    4. Evaluation

44. That which distinguishes one job from all others is the job _____. (*p. 149*)
    1. Specification
    2. Description
    3. Title
    4. Evaluation

45. A coordinated and aggregated series of work elements used to produce an output, for example, making a bed, is known as a _____. (*p. 149*)
    1. Job specification
    2. Job description
    3. Task
    4. Job evaluation

46. The administrator asks the financial manager to identify competition for personnel, estimate in-migration or out-migration of workers, and look at wage scales in the area. The administrator wants _____. (*p. 150*)
    1. An orientation to the area
    2. A job family to be established
    3. A person power inventory
    4. More information than is needed

47. The authority of government agencies to review facility recruitment sources, advertising and statistics on the number of applicants, and persons hired by category stems from _____. (*p. 152*)
    1. The Americans With Disabilities Act
    2. The Equal Opportunities Commission
    3. The Civil Rights Act
    4. New federal powers

48. The geographical scope of a search for applicants for a nursing assistant or housekeeping job is likely to be limited to _____. (*p. 153*)
    1. The state
    2. Commuting distance
    3. The county
    4. That region of the United States

49. Present employees, career ladders, job posting, and job bidding are _____. (*p. 153*)
    1. Inappropriate recruiting sources
    2. Good recruiting sources
    3. Too expensive as recruiting sources
    4. Unrelated to the applicant pool

50. Career ladders are paths along which the employee _____. (*p. 153*)
    1. Finds limitations
    2. Is restricted
    3. Finds unlimited options
    4. Can hope to progress

51. Posting a job opening on the facility bulletin board is _____. (*pp. 153–154*)
    1. Generally a good practice
    2. Required by the Equal Employment Opportunities Commission (EEOC)
    3. Required by the Civil Rights Act
    4. Poor personnel practice

52. Use of a search firm would be more appropriate for hiring a _____. (*p. 155*)
    1. New director of activities
    2. Well-qualified nurse
    3. New administrator
    4. Registered dietitian

2.6 HIRING STAFF

53. Recruitment is the process of _____ prospective staff. (*p. 157*)
    1. Locating
    2. Screening
    3. Interviewing
    4. Placing

54. Personnel selection is the process of _____. (*p. 157*)
    1. Deciding which applicant best fits the job requirements
    2. Setting up interviews with applicants
    3. Reviewing interview results
    4. Hiring and firing

55. Prohibiting discrimination on the basis of race, color, religion, sex, or national origin is the basis of the _____. (*p. 157*)
    1. Wagner Act
    2. Civil Legislation Act
    3. Employment Act
    4. Civil Rights Act

56. The Civil Rights Act Title 7 and the Equal Employment Act of 1972 apply to employers of _____ or more employees. (*p. 158*)
    1. 50
    2. 100
    3. 200
    4. 15

57. The employer interviews 90 Black applicants and 30 White applicants, then hires 30 White and 30 Black applicants. If applicants were hired in these proportions over time, the facility would likely experience _____. (*p. 158*)
    1. Reverse impact
    2. Reverse discrimination
    3. Worker pool depletion
    4. Adverse impact

58. The staff development coordinator sent a candidate to five different department heads who used the newly developed application form and obtained the same score results. The staff development coordinator can reasonably feel that the application form has _____. (*p. 159*)
    1. Reasonable reliability
    2. Good validity
    3. A great future
    4. Construct validity

59. The staff development coordinator asks several of the department heads if the application form the coordinator has developed is helping them match candidates with job descriptions. The coordinator is wondering if the instrument has _____. (*p. 160*)
    1. Content validity
    2. Reliability
    3. Usefulness
    4. Repeatability

60. The staff development coordinator has found an instrument that measures a trait believed important to jobs in nursing facilities. The staff development coordinator believes this instrument has _____. (*p. 160*)
    1. Construct validity
    2. Reliability
    3. Definite usefulness
    4. Content validity

61. The director of nursing asks an job applicant's age and religious affiliation. This is _____. (*p. 160*)
    1. Illegal
    2. Encouraged
    3. Necessary to the interview
    4. Permissible under certain circumstances

62. After hiring an applicant, the staff development coordinator demands that the new hire bring in a photograph or allow one to be made at the facility. This is _____. (*p. 161*)
    1. Illegal
    2. Legal
    3. Necessary to the interview
    4. Permissible under certain circumstances

63. The director of nursing asks whether an applicant nurse is willing to work on Easter. This is _____. (*p. 162*)
    1. Illegal
    2. Legal
    3. Necessary to the interview
    4. Permissible under certain circumstances

64. The director of nursing asks the nurse candidate how much alcohol she consumes per week. This is _____. (*p. 163*)
    1. Illegal
    2. Legal
    3. Necessary to the interview
    4. Permissible under certain circumstances

65. The director of nursing asks the applicant whether he has ever been treated for drug problems. This is _____. (*p. 163*)
    1. Illegal
    2. Legal
    3. Necessary to the interview
    4. Permissible under certain circumstances

66. The director of nursing asks the treatment nurse applicant a predetermined and set array of questions. The director of nursing is using a/an _____ interview approach. (*p. 164*)
    1. Nondirective
    2. Directive
    3. In-depth
    4. Patterned

67. A director of nursing asking a nurse supervisor applicant, "What actions have you taken if you disagreed with a supervisor's decision?" is _____. (*p. 164*)
    1. Illegal
    2. Legal
    3. Necessary to the interview
    4. Permissible under certain circumstances

68. Research results suggest that interviews for job applicants may be better for explaining _____. (*p. 165*)
    1. Why a person would not be a good candidate
    2. Why a person is a good candidate
    3. What truly motivates the applicant
    4. The applicant's true value system

69. When asked, an applicant reveals that she has been convicted in an area relevant to the job being sought. The director of nursing then considers the nature, number, facts surrounding, job-relatedness, and length of time since or between convictions. This is _____. (*p. 166*)
    1. Illegal
    2. Legal
    3. Necessary to the interview
    4. Permissible under certain circumstances

70. Credit reports on job applicants _____. (*p. 166*)
    1. Require the applicant's permission
    2. Are routinely done
    3. Are usually not meaningful
    4. Are illegal

71. A good risk management-related reason for requiring a physical examination before any new employee begins work is to _____. (*p. 167*)
    1. Discover any handicaps
    2. Be able to assess the employee's future health needs
    3. Be able to inform relevant staff of any limitations
    4. Provide a baseline against which to assess later exams or claims

72. If the physician determines that the new employee cannot perform essential functions of the position accepted due to a disability covered under the Americans With Disabilities Act, the facility _____. (*p. 167*)
    1. Must assist in finding placement in another facility
    2. Must make a reasonable accommodation
    3. Inform the applicant of unsuitability
    4. Put the new hire to work in the position for which he or she was hired

73. In most nursing facilities, the final decision to hire a job applicant is made by the _____. (p. 169)
    1. Director of personnel
    2. Staff development coordinator
    3. Administrator
    4. Department head

74. Thirty years ago, successful caring for the frail elderly in the facility often depended less on technical knowledge than compassion for others. Today, successful caring for the frail elderly in the facility increasingly depends on _____. (p. 169)
    1. Technical knowledge
    2. Even more compassion
    3. Both technical knowledge and compassion
    4. Ability to perform the job specifications

75. Nurses and nursing assistants who have drive and enthusiasm for caring for the patient _____. (p. 170)
    1. Have everything necessary
    2. Have the essential ingredients
    3. Can be taught technical skills they lack
    4. Have a reduced role in the modern facility

76. Applicants who lack fire in their hearts or passion for their work are _____. (p. 170)
    1. Relatively easy to "fire up"
    2. Are not so easily taught these attributes
    3. Need to be technically competent to compensate
    4. Are still good candidates if technically competent

77. The hiring decision itself _____. (p. 169)
    1. Is complex
    2. Takes care of itself
    3. Is usually clear
    4. Should be done based on numbers

2.7 TRAINING STAFF

78. The first day on the job _____. (p. 171)
    1. Is usually a blur
    2. Is less important than later
    3. Leaves a lasting impression
    4. Produces little output

79. Official welcome, introduction to staff, and a tour of the facility are activities best associated with the _____. (*p. 172*)
    1. First week on the job
    2. Pre-job visit
    3. First day on the job
    4. Orientation, at some point

80. Valuable tax credits can be achieved if the facility ensures that employees comply with the _____. (*pp. 172–173*)
    1. Civil Rights Acts requirements
    2. Americans With Disabilities Act
    3. Tax credit for handicapped workers
    4. Targeted Jobs Tax Credit Program

81. A compilation of facility policies that directly relate to work conditions is _____. (*p. 172*)
    1. The employee contract
    2. The preemployment orientation
    3. A legal agreement between employer and employee
    4. The employee handbook

82. Employers who have entered clear disclaimers in the employee handbook have _____ successful employee suits in court alleging the handbook to be a binding contract. (*p. 174*)
    1. Prevented
    2. Encouraged
    3. Proliferated
    4. Not prevented

83. When the staff development coordinator reviews job descriptions and the activities essential for performing each job, the coordinator is performing a _____. (*p. 175*)
    1. Service to the facility
    2. Needed personnel action
    3. Task analysis
    4. Employee skills analysis

84. Employee education offered throughout the work career of the employee, often of a mandatory nature, is typically referred to as _____. (*p. 175*)
    1. Skill sharpening
    2. Continuing education
    3. Seminars
    4. Inservice training

85. One way to improve evaluation of training efforts is to state learning objectives
_____. (*p. 176*)
   1. As learning objectives
   2. As objectively as possible
   3. In quantifiable terms
   4. As behavioral objectives

2.8 RETAINING EMPLOYEES

86. Social approval, self-esteem, security, and use of power are examples of _____.
(*p. 178*)
   1. What employers seek from employees
   2. What each employer offers employees
   3. What employees seek from the facility
   4. Overly idealistic goals

87. Generally, if the community or significant others disapprove of the employee
working at a facility, the employee _____. (*p. 178*)
   1. Will quit
   2. Will redouble efforts
   3. Not have positive feelings about working at the facility
   4. Will be enabled by facility attitude to ignore this

88. Being part of a facility that has a sense of purpose to which an employee can
dedicate energy with pride enhances an employee's _____. (*p. 178*)
   1. Merit pay expectations
   2. Sense of destiny
   3. Willingness to volunteer
   4. Self-esteem

89. Employees who are enjoying a high level of job satisfaction are more likely to
_____. (*p. 179*)
   1. Require additional benefits
   2. Attend significant in-service training sessions
   3. Achieve educational goals
   4. Provide a high level of patient care

90. Employees want to work for an employer who _____. (*p. 179*)
   1. Pays outstanding stock dividends
   2. Has a AAA rating in the market
   3. Has a great education program
   4. Stimulates their dreams and aspirations

91. Among the following, the most important needs of the staff from the administrator is to _____. (*p. 179*)
    1. Provide a large array of educational options
    2. Ensure that the bonuses are distributed equitably
    3. Meet their self-actuating needs
    4. Take a personal interest in them

92. Every day, administrators in more than 16,000 nursing facilities make personnel decisions based on _____. (*p. 179*)
    1. What they were taught in personnel class
    2. The psychologist they most admire
    3. The theories they have read and assimilated
    4. Their assumptions of what motivates the staff

93. The assumptions that employees naturally dislike work, prefer to receive extensive direction from superiors, and work to avoid responsibility characterize the _____. (*p. 180*)
    1. Human relations school
    2. Scientific management school
    3. Theory X philosophy
    4. Theory Y philosophy

94. Managers who believe that using energy to work is as natural as using energy to play or rest, that individuals can exercise self-direction, and that individuals seek and accept responsibility accept the approach characterized as the _____. (*p. 180*)
    1. Human relations school
    2. Scientific management school
    3. Theory X philosophy
    4. Theory Y philosophy

95. A test often used by facility personnel staff that has 100 questions asking respondents how they feel or act in a variety of situations, then places respondents into categories of introverted or extroverted, sensing or intuitive, thinking or feeling, and perceiving or judging is the _____. (*p. 181*)
    1. Complete Personality Analyses Series
    2. Myers–Briggs Type Indicator
    3. Left-brain, right-brain analysis
    4. Simpsons Personality Series

96. Persons characterized as systematic, thorough, and balanced and who ask detailed questions about each situation are characterized as _____. (*p. 181*)
    1. Right brained
    2. Left brained
    3. Influenced
    4. Balanced

97. Persons characterized as more intuitive, quick, and less complex in their approach to decision making are characterized as _____. (*p. 181*)
    1. Right brained
    2. Left brained
    3. Influenced
    4. Balanced

98. One safer generalization about employee motives is that _____. (*p. 182*)
    1. They are predictable
    2. They are always mixed
    3. Little is known about them
    4. They are manageable

99. Some motives/needs may recede when satisfied, for example, hunger or thirst; other motives such as the need for power _____. (*p. 182*)
    1. Follow the same pattern
    2. Are unpredictable
    3. Disappear when met
    4. May become more intensified when partially achieved

100. The process of giving employees increased roles in the decision-making processes of the facility is sometimes called _____. (*p. 182*)
    1. Overuse of resources
    2. Underuse of management authority and direction
    3. Division of power
    4. Job enrichment

101. In Maslow's hierarchy of needs concept, it is _____ to meet lower needs before higher needs become salient. (*p. 182*)
    1. Necessary
    2. Easy
    3. Incorrect
    4. Optional

102. Employees who are hard driving and achievement oriented and who strive constantly to achieve higher levels are characterized as _____. (*p. 183*)
    1. Type A
    2. Type B
    3. Driven
    4. Successful

103. Persons who have only moderate achievement needs, are less competitive, and more satisfied with moderation whether in sports, titles, or on-the-job productivity are characterized as _____. (*p. 184*)
    1. Type A
    2. Type B
    3. Less driven
    4. Cool

104. In the nursing facility setting, _____ persons are required to be either certified or licensed. (*p. 185*)
1. Nearly all
2. About half
3. Nearly two thirds
4. Few

105. When a patient wanders away, walks away, runs away, escapes, or otherwise leaves a caregiving facility or environment unsupervised, unnoticed, and/or before the scheduled discharge, the patient has _____. (*pp. 121–122*)
1. Gone back home
2. Wandered into the street
3. Eloped
4. Found care at the facility to be wanting

106. A charge nurse being encouraged to become a nurse practitioner and a nurse's aide being supported to seek to become a licensed practical nurse are examples of a facility commitment to provide employees _____. (*p. 185*)
1. Good chance to get ahead
2. Upward mobility
3. More education
4. A career path

107. Pain is _____. (*p. 123*)
1. Often overtreated
2. Seldom treated
3. What the patient says it is
4. Impossible to measure

108. The most reliable indicator of pain is _____. (*p. 123*)
1. Facial expression
2. Seen in the eyes
3. When a resident winces on movement
4. The resident's self-report

109. Employees prefer to work in a facility in which mistakes _____. (*p. 186*)
1. Are not emphasized
2. Are forgiven
3. Are expected
4. Are kept from harming anyone

110. The medication nurse who bursts into the director of nursing's office and bemoans making a 20% error rate on her last attempt to pass medications has _____. (*p. 186*)
1. Put the facility into jeopardy
2. Failed to do reasonable risk management
3. Really messed up
4. Set the stage for communication and improvement

111. The idea that when reward follows performance, performance improves and that when rewards do not follow performance, performance deteriorates is known as _____. (*p. 186*)
    1. Expectancy theory
    2. Reward theory
    3. Reinforcement theory
    4. A flawed approach

112. The reduction in degrees of freedom in decision making brought about by well-developed policies is _____. (*p. 187*)
    1. Always a plus
    2. The crux of a good risk-management program
    3. A potential downside of having good policies
    4. The conformity it is necessary to ensure

113. Department heads who conform are defensive, produce detailed substantiation of unimportant problems, and give invalid information illustrate _____. (*p. 187*)
    1. Argyris's belief that organizations tend to treat employees as immature
    2. That organizations need good communication channels
    3. Today's organizations
    4. How they may actually be helping the organization

114. The idea of treating each employee as a member of the team is _____. (*p. 188*)
    1. An unrealistic goal
    2. Not functional in a nursing facility setting
    3. An effort to combat powerlessness, to give employees "ownership"
    4. Always effective

115. A director of nursing who consults aides about whether they are prepared to receive a new admission and acts on the aides' decision is an attempt to _____. (*p. 189*)
    1. Give ownership to the aides and treat them as "business persons"
    2. Be sensitive to the aides' work loads
    3. Get advice from all sources
    4. Be a good communicator

116. One of the major tasks of the administrator is to _____. (*p. 189*)
    1. Treat employees civilly
    2. Be supportive of employees needs
    3. Create and enforce opportunities for staff to feel in control
    4. Create opportunities for staff to vent their feelings

117. High patient care depends, in part, on whether the administrator is able to _____. (*p. 190*)
     1. Reward staff sufficiently
     2. Defend staff to residents and families
     3. Create career ladders for all staff
     4. Enable the employees to "buy" into the facility

118. "It'll never work," "we've tried that 20 times already," "yes, but…" are common responses to new suggestions known as _____. (*p. 190*)
     1. Negation
     2. Not invented here
     3. Circular nature of organizations
     4. Fire hoses

119. Somatic, visceral, and bone are _____. (*p. 123*)
     1. Categories of pain
     2. Precursors of pain
     3. Independent of pain
     4. Generally untreatable pain

120. Abuse, neglect, superficial/substantial injuries of unknown source, misappropriated property _____. (*p. 204*)
     1. Are an unfortunate reality
     2. Must be reduced
     3. Must be prevented
     4. Must be reported to authorities

121. A good rule of thumb in the treatment of pain is to _____. (*pp. 123–124*)
     1. Treat fully
     2. Treat aggressively
     3. Use several drugs
     4. Use lowest effective dose

2.9 EVALUATING EMPLOYEES

122. There are those, such as Deming, who argue that being the member of a productive team affords the facility managers sufficient evaluation and control over employee's performance. One potential problem with this is that _____. (*p. 194*)
     1. It fosters team membership
     2. It stifles creativity
     3. Organizations' memories are short
     4. Employees like to have written records of their work

123. Job performance evaluation is intended to be a function of comparing and controlling personnel _____. (*p. 194*)
    1. Attitudes
    2. Approaches to management
    3. Behavior
    4. Performance quality

124. The absence of any written system for evaluation of long-term performance exposes the individual more nearly to _____. (*p. 195*)
    1. Good judgment of current managers
    2. Evaluation on present work
    3. Higher appraisals
    4 The whim of managers

125. Employees, it has been observed, normally _____. (*p. 195*)
    1. Outperform their self-image
    2. Do not outperform their self-image
    3. Are self-starting, for the most part
    4. Require little supervision in the traditional nursing facility setting

126. An evaluator checking off the extent to which an employee meets a trait or requirement is using a/an _____. (*p. 196*)
    1. Outmoded model
    2. Performance scale
    3. Rating scale
    4. Global rating

127. Department heads who consistently give high ratings to avoid conflict illustrate the _____. (*p. 196*)
    1. Abuse of global ratings
    2. Leniency error
    3. Error of central tendency
    4. Halo effect

128. The supervisor is impressed by the fact that the employee never missed a day and was never late, so rated the employee highly overall. This is a(an) _____. (*p. 196*)
    1. Abuse of global ratings
    2. Leniency error
    3. Error of central tendency
    4. Halo effect

129. Transfer, promotion, demotion, and layoff are possible outcomes of _____. (*p. 197*)
    1. Poor work attitudes
    2. A performance appraisal
    3. Good rating scales at work
    4. Global ratings for some managers

2.10 PAYING EMPLOYEES

130. Workers expecting an exchange in which their wages and benefits are equal to their work effort when compared with similarly situated employees illustrate the _____. (*pp. 199–200*)
    1. Resiliency of worker expectation
    2. Fair exchange theory
    3. Compensation theory
    4. Equity theory

131. Giving an across-the-board wage increase based on the Consumer Price Index is giving a(an) _____. (*p. 201*)
    1. Well-deserved raise to the staff
    2. Boost in staff pay levels
    3. Cost of living increase
    4. Indexed wage increase

132. In the nursing facility, the key job against which many staff measure their wages is compensation of the _____. (*p. 202*)
    1. Administrator
    2. Medical director
    3. Owner
    4. Director of nursing

2.11 DISCIPLINING EMPLOYEES

133. Unless the facility can convincingly illustrate that it had a "just cause" for firing an employee, that employee will likely _____. (*p. 203*)
    1. Be rehired
    2. Remain on the facility payroll
    3. Collect unemployment
    4. Complain to the state

134. Grievance procedures offer a needed _____. (*p. 203*)
    1. Source of discipline
    2. Safety valve
    3. Protection to the management
    4. Reciprocity relationship

135. With the ultrasound stethoscope, the nursing facility nurse will be providing ___-like monitoring in the nursing facility setting. (*p. 126*)
    1. Home health care
    2. Doctor's office
    3. Emergency department
    4. Intensive care unit

136. Lean body mass and bone mineral contents usually _____ with age. (*p. 130*)
1. Increase
2. Decrease
3. Disappear
4. Melt

137. A decrease in intestinal motility characteristically accompanies _____. (*p. 131*)
1. Poor diet
2. Reduced food intake
3. Overeating
4. Aging

138. Succeeding in caregiving includes communicating the facility's care efforts to both the resident and the _____ surrounding each resident. (*p. 143*)
1. Roommates
2. Hall maters
3. Suite mates
4. Support networks

139. An increasing amount of valuable personnel information can be obtained through using smart _____. (*p. 177*)
1. ID badges
2. Videos
3. Audios
4. Cameras on every hall

NAB Domain: Finance/Business

Learning to Manage the Organization's Finances

1. The staff person responsible for ensuring that the business office runs smoothly is, in the final analysis, _____. (*p. 210*)*
   1. Corporate finance director
   2. The administrator
   3. Business office staff
   4. Facility treasurer

2. In general, the ownership patterns for U.S. nursing facilities in 2006 _____. (*p. 211*)
   1. Were unstable
   2. Varied widely from state to state
   3. Were somewhat stable
   4. Were unchanged from 89 years earlier

3. Generating reports on the financial standing of the nursing facility is generally assigned to _____. (*p. 210*)
   1. The accountant
   2. The director of finance
   3. The administrative assistant
   4. The chief financial officer (CFO)

4. Responsibility and blame for overspending in the department of nursing and in food services are typically assigned by the owners to the _____. (*p. 211*)
   1. Director of nursing and director of food services
   2. Director of nursing and the dietitian
   3. Chief financial officer
   4. Administrator

---

*Answers can be found in *Nursing Home Administration*, Seventh Edition, on the page numbers in parentheses following each question.

5. A set of records that lists each monetary transaction of the facility is normally referred to as _____. (*p. 213*)
   1. The books
   2. Financial statements
   3. Monetary records
   4. Income and revenue statement

6. The primary purpose of the Generally Accepted Accounting Principles is to _____. (*p. 213*)
   1. Guarantee honesty among providers
   2. Maximize comparability of financial statements of different organizations
   3. Create a single view among financial managers
   4. Protect the owners

7. An owner who takes unrecorded cash from the facility's daily cash intake to purchase a tablet for his daughter to use at college has violated the _____ concept. (*p. 213*)
   1. Consistency
   2. Entity
   3. Time period
   4. Objective evidence

8. Instructing the financial manager to record assets at current market value and to not record patient bills expected to become uncollectible violates the _____ concept. (*p. 214*)
   1. Entity
   2. Good faith
   3. Time period
   4. Consistency

9. Telling the accountant not to record overtime paid from the cash box to employees working weekends is violating the _____ concept. (*p. 214*)
   1. Ongoing concern
   2. Entity
   3. Full disclosure
   4. Time period

10. Directing the accountant to move from a January 1 date to a June 30 fiscal year date in order to minimize the negative image possibly created by an anticipated loss violates the _____ concept. (*p. 214*)
    1. Ongoing concern
    2. Time period
    3. Conservation
    4. Entity

11. Allowing the bookkeeper to destroy vouchers showing payments made for meals to employees once these are recorded may violate the _____ concept. (*p. 214*)
    1. Objective evidence
    2. Consistency
    3. Time period
    4. Entity

12. Pieces of paper indicating money owed to or by the facility, bank statements, and similar pieces of paper or their electronic equivalents are known as _____. (*p. 214*)
    1. Paper trail
    2. Source documents
    3. Bill of lading
    4. Records

13. An administrator who instructs the accountant to begin reporting facility finances by recording all expenditures and all receipts as they actually occur has decided to use the _____ system of accounting. (*p. 216*)
    1. Cash
    2. Implied
    3. No-fault
    4. Accrual

14. It is difficult to recognize items such as depreciation and prepaid insurance in the _____ system of accounting. (*p. 216*)
    1. Accrual
    2. Simplified
    3. Cash
    4. Income and expense

15. An administrator directing the accountant to record revenues when they are earned and expenses when they are incurred regardless of the time the cash transaction takes place has decided to use the _____ approach to accounting. (*p. 216*)
    1. Accrual
    2. Cash
    3. Simplified
    4. Advanced

16. Allowing the facility to accurately measure revenues earned after expenses have been paid or losses incurred by matching revenues and expenses for each time period is the advantage of the _____ system of accounting. (*p. 216*)
    1. Accrual
    2. Cash
    3. Income and loss
    4. Advanced electronic

17. A summary of the nursing home's financial well-being within a time period is normally referred to as _____. (*p. 217*)
    1. The financial statements
    2. Profit and loss
    3. Notes to changes in financial condition
    4. Statements of change

18. If the administrator asked the bookkeeper for a list containing every account in the facility, the bookkeeper would hand the administrator the _____. (*p. 217*)
    1. Books
    2. Financial report
    3. Chart of accounts
    4. General journal

19. Things owned by the facility are normally referred to as _____. (*p. 217*)
    1. Debentures
    2. Assets
    3. Possessions
    4. Tangibles

20. Things owed by the facility, its obligations, are normally referred to as _____. (*p. 217*)
    1. Capital
    2. Unpaid bills
    3. Invoices
    4. Liabilities

21. Money invested in the facility, also known as the facility's net worth, is normally referred to as _____. (*p. 218*)
    1. Stock
    2. Collateral
    3. Capital
    4. Income stream

22. If the administrator asks the accountant for the journals, the administrator wants to look at _____. (*p. 218*)
    1. The original entries
    2. The assets
    3. The debits
    4. Current summaries of income and outgo

23. The new accountant informs the administrator that to simplify things, he has incorporated all purchases that will be paid for the next few years into the accounts payable journal. The administrator should _____. (*p. 218*)
    1. Compliment the accountant
    2. Ask for last year's books to be conformed to the new system
    3. Begin a search for a new accountant
    4. Ask that these purchases be transferred to the general journal

24. Making a debit and a credit entry for each transaction is known as the _____ system of accounting. (*p. 218*)
    1. Single/double
    2. Systematic
    3. Alternate
    4. Double-entry

25. Under double-entry bookkeeping, when a bill is sent to Ms. Jones for $3,000 for the past month's care, the bookkeeper would normally record $3,000 in the debit column as an increase in assets and _____. (*p. 221*)
    1. Record $3,000 on the credit side as an increase in revenue
    2. Record $3,000 as received
    3. Wait for the payment before entering further data
    4. Enter an estimate of when the bill will be paid

26. Using accrual accounting, purchase of a 6-month supply of provisions would be entered into the _____. (*p. 221*)
    1. Billings journal
    2. Cash receipts journal
    3. General journal
    4. Credit side of the ledger

27. Under accrual accounting, when the accountant shows the amount of medical supplies used during a month in the cash disbursements journal and the general journal, the bookkeeper has made _____. (*p. 222*)
    1. A mistake
    2. An adjusting entry
    3. An inappropriate entry
    4. A good accounting judgment

28. When errors are discovered in other journals, they can be corrected by entries into the _____. (*p. 222*)
    1. Support records
    2. Ledger
    3. Cash receipts journal
    4. General journal

29. When the administrator asks the accountant for a summary of all debits and credits contained in the journals for the time period, the accountant should hand the _____ to the administrator. (*p. 222*)
    1. General journal
    2. General ledger
    3. Financial statements
    4. Debits and credits listing

30. At the end of a time period, when debits do not match credits exactly, the accountant can first assume that an error has been made in _____. (*p. 223*)
    1. Recording transactions
    2. Entering debits
    3. Entering credits
    4. Source documents

31. The Generally Accepted Accounting Principles (GAAP) do not normally require financial statements prepared for general distribution to include _____. (*p. 224*)
    1. Income statement, or profit/loss statement
    2. Balance sheet, or statement of financial position
    3. Statement of changes in financial position
    4. Chart of accounts

32. The income statement shows whether _____ were sufficient to cover expenses. (*p. 224*)
    1. Charges
    2. Revenues
    3. Debts
    4. Retained earnings

33. The accountant has listed the new building annex, the new central air conditioning system, and the supplies for the next 6 months as capital expenses. The administrator should _____. (*p. 224*)
    1. Be pleased with the decisions
    2. Forward the report to corporate headquarters
    3. Rewrite the report
    4. Look for a new accountant

34. At the end of a time period, total expenses are subtracted from total revenues to compute the _____. (*p. 227*)
    1. Net income, or profit or loss
    2. Approximate income
    3. Adjusted income margin
    4. Operating income

35. The accountant, upon successfully bringing the expense and revenue accounts to zero, has successfully _____. (*p. 227*)
    1. Calculated profit
    2. Calculated losses
    3. Closed the books
    4. Completed the financial statements

36. When the administrator asks the chief financial officer (CFO) for a statement showing the ending balance of the revenue and expense accounts, the CFO should hand the _____ to the administrator. (*p. 227*)
    1. Income statement
    2. Balance sheet
    3. General ledger
    4. General journal

37. A financial statement in which the assets must equal the liability and capital accounts is known as the _____. (*p. 227*)
    1. Ending statement
    2. Final statement
    3. Balance sheet
    4. Financial statement

38. Any possession of the facility that will be or could be turned into cash within 12 months is a _____. (*p. 227*)
    1. Noncurrent asset
    2. Current asset
    3. Benefit
    4. Positive asset

39. Because capital assets will not be liquidated any time soon, their current market value is not directly relevant relates to the ongoing concern concept and is known as _____. (*p. 229*)
    1. Historic cost
    2. Current cost
    3. Original cost
    4. Projected value

40. Depreciation is an expense associated with the use of _____. (*p. 229*)
    1. A purchase
    2. An asset
    3. Land
    4. A specified purchase

41. Bills from suppliers of foodstuffs or office supplies or janitorial services contractors are normally classified as among the _____. (*p. 229*)
1. Current liabilities
2. Accounts due
3. Invoices
4. Bills of lading

42. When an administrator notes that there are $600,000 in notes payable on the financial reports, the administrator knows these must be paid within _____. (*p. 229*)
1. 6 months
2. 1 year
3. 1 month
4. 90 days

43. Funds that have been put into the facility by owners or others, and retained earnings that have been put back into the facility are usually included when calculating the _____. (*p. 229*)
1. Net worth
2. Bottom line
3. Final value
4. Financial liabilities

44. Except for for-profit facilities paying taxes and the not-for-profit facility not paying income taxes, there are_____ in accounting and financial processes. (*p. 224*)
1. Only a few significant differences
2. No real differences
3. No real similarities
4. Increasingly fewer similarities

45. Not having to pay taxes gives not-for-profit facilities a slight _____. (*p. 224*)
1. Disadvantage
2. A competitive edge
3. Increase in more incentives
4. A large investment opportunities

46. The certified public accountant's end-of-year report for a 15-year-old 120-bed for-profit facility with no debt shows an excess of income over expenses of $95,000. The owners would likely be _____. (*p. 230*)
1. Very pleased with facility performance
2. Very displeased with facility performance
3. Generally satisfied
4. Neutral

47. When asked whether funds are readily available for a $75,000 purchase and the accountant responds that the net worth is well over $800,000 and to go ahead with the purchase, the administrator should _____. (*p. 231*)
    1. Ask for a statement of working capital
    2. Make the purchase
    3. Seek a vertical analysis
    4. Amortize the purchase

48. When the amount of current assets remaining after current liabilities have been subtracted is calculated, the administrator has an idea of the _____ available to be spent. (*p. 231*)
    1. Capital
    2. Net worth
    3. Working capital
    4. Assets

49. When the CFO identifies trends in measures of financial performance of the facility by comparing the same relationships for several time periods he is doing _____. (*p. 232*)
    1. Comparison analyses
    2. Time period analyses
    3. Ratio analyses
    4. Trade-off comparisons

50. A facility has current assets of $403,898 and current liabilities of $367,000. Its current ratio is _____. (*p. 232*)
    1. 9
    2. 3
    3. 1.1
    4. 2.1

51. A 1-year-old, 120-bed for-profit facility with a $2,500,000 mortgage at 7.4% reports a net operating margin before depreciation of $25,000. In today's financial market, the owners would likely be _____. (*p. 234*)
    1. Very pleased
    2. Very displeased
    3. Seeking to sell the facility as a result
    4. Seeking to refinance as a result

52. Ratios, to be truly useful, should be _____. (*p. 232*)
    1. Used to measure over time
    2. Compared with industry averages over time
    3. In simple mathematical terms
    4. Compared to expected future ratios

53. The new administrator in a private pay for-profit facility is told by the accountant that the accounts receivable are $105,800 and the net operating revenues are $334,000. On calculating the average collection period ratio, which turns out to be _____ days, the administrator should be _____. (*p. 234*)
    1. 29/pleased
    2. 20/displeased
    3. 115/pleased
    4. 115/upset

54. A 12-year-old facility, largely out of debt, has $334,693 in operating revenues and $339,078 in operating expenses, yielding a net operating margin ratio of _____. The owners of this facility would likely feel this to be _____. (*p. 234*)
    1. 0.013/unacceptable
    2. 0.013/acceptable
    3. 8.013/unacceptable
    4. 8.013/acceptable

55. A facility with long-term debt of $4,000,000 and a total equity of $3,000,000 has a debt-to-equity ratio of _____, which is _____ the industry average. (*p. 234*)
    1. 1.33/considerably above
    2. 1.33/considerably below
    3. 2.33/far above
    4. 2.33/well below

56. Trends and patterns in the operation of a nursing facility can best be obtained by doing _____. (*p. 236*)
    1. Ratio analyses
    2. Vertical analyses
    3. Ratio and vertical analyses over time
    4. Ratio and vertical analyses

57. To safeguard the finances of a facility, procedures should be arranged to establish a system of _____ so that employees review each other's financial activities. (*p. 238*)
    1. Checks
    2. Dual bookkeeping
    3. Checks and balances
    4. Antitheft devices

58. A useful form that summarizes the facility's occupancy, listing daily admissions, discharges, and transfers is known as the _____. (*p. 239*)
    1. Daily census form
    2. Headcount
    3. Weekly census report
    4. Occupancy ratio

59. At the end of each year for facilities participating in Medicare, a Medicare Cost Reconciliation settlement occurs, in which _____. (*p. 245*)
1. The facility receives additional money
2. The facility pays out additional money
3. The facility receives or pays back money
4. A flat rate per patient per month is paid the facility

60. The frozen food contractor arrives, places the order in the freezer, checks off the receiving slip, hands it to the appropriate kitchen employee who thanks the contractor and hands the receiving slip and purchase order copy to the director of food services. The administrator, on observing this, should _____. (*p. 246*)
1. Be pleased with the smoothness of the working relationship
2. Compliment the contractor for an efficient delivery
3. Be upset
4. Continue to enjoy his or her cup of coffee

61. Perhaps the only way to maintain an accurate count of supplies consumed and those remaining is to use _____. (*p. 250*)
1. A computer program
2. A hand-counted inventory system
3. A receipt inventory system
4. A perpetual inventory system

62. The use of LIFO (last in/first out) to price inventory during a period of inflation will have the effect of making the value of the goods remaining in inventory _____. (*p. 251*)
1. Higher
2. Lower
3. About the same
4. At market value

63. The largest directly controllable cost for the average administrator is _____. (*p. 252*)
1. Inventory/supplies
2. Labor
3. Long-term debt financing costs
4. Short-term debt financing costs

64. Payroll deductions are subtracted from _____ to arrive at the employee's _____ pay. (*p. 252*)
1. Net/gross
2. Total/net
3. Gross/net
4. Overall/take home

65. Assets that can be capitalized or depreciated differ from the other assets of a facility in that they are used in operations for more than _____ and will not be converted into _____ within the year. (*p. 256*)
    1. One time period/cash
    2. Two time periods/debt
    3. A balance sheet period/securities
    4. Three years/cash

66. On discovering that the new accountant had set the actual purchase price paid (e.g., no tax, delivery, or similar costs) for the assets to be depreciated, the facility administrator would normally feel the accountant was _____. (*p. 256*)
    1. Sharp and on the ball
    2. Not serving the facility well
    3. Overestimating historical costs
    4. Doing okay, all things considered

67. One practical reason for using straight line depreciation is that _____. (*p. 257*)
    1. It brings the fastest write-off
    2. It is the only fully acceptable method
    3. Most third-party payers require it
    4. It has the approval of the Internal Revenue Service (IRS)

68. Congress' purpose for passing accelerated depreciation was to _____ of new facilities. (*p. 257*)
    1. Discourage overbuilding
    2. Encourage more building
    3. Regulate construction
    4. Deregulate construction

69. As a practical matter, most owners do not fund depreciation and treat it as _____. (*p. 258*)
    1. Money available to the facility to spend
    2. Money to be placed in reserve
    3. A fiction
    4. A useless set of required calculations

70. Using several differing depreciation schedules for a single piece of equipment is _____ as an accounting behavior. (*p. 259*)
    1. Unacceptable
    2. Quite acceptable
    3. Risky
    4. Illegal

71. Land _____ is a depreciable asset. (*p. 229*)
    1. Never
    2. Sometimes
    3. For for-profit facilities
    4. For nonprofit facilities

72. Medical supplies, food supplies, and postage for billing residents are _____ costs. (*p. 260*)
    1. Fixed
    2. Variable
    3. Semi-variable
    4. Break-even

73. The salary of the director of nursing and the administrator are examples of _____ costs. (*p. 260*)
    1. Fixed
    2. Variable
    3. Semi-variable
    4. Proportionate

74. In a facility having high fixed costs the pressure to keep beds filled is _____ in facilities with low fixed costs. (*p. 261*)
    1. About the same as
    2. Stronger than
    3. Weaker than
    4. More moderate than

75. For in-facility services such as physical therapy it is important to calculate the _____ cost in order to better analyze the cost-effectiveness of such services. (*p. 262*)
    1. Total
    2. Break-even
    3. Minimum
    4. Maximum

76. Nursing and physical therapy are normally thought of as _____ centers. (*p. 262*)
    1. Cost
    2. Loss
    3. Revenue
    4. Break-even

77. A financial analysis that yields to the administrator a representative picture of the entire expense of providing a service (e.g., offering adult day care services) is known as _____. (*p. 264*)
    1. Value analysis
    2. Revenue analysis
    3. Cost finding
    4. Center analysis

78. Only when appropriate _____ has been achieved can an accurate job of _____be accomplished. (*p. 265*)
1. Information/gathering cost setting
2. Cost finding/rate setting
3. Expense reporting/estimating income
4. Tax analysis/cost setting

79. In order to develop a reasonable estimate of income and expenses for a coming time period it is important to do both a(an) _____ budget and a _____ budget. (*p. 270*)
1. Capital/cash
2. Expense/revenue
3. Expense/balanced
4. Cash/capital

80. Because income and expenses vary from time period to time period, it is desirable to project a _____ budget. (*p. 272*)
1. Cash
2. Balanced
3. Forecasted
4. Capital

81. Plans for expenditures for buildings, major equipment, and the like are normally part of the _____ budget. (*p. 273*)
1. Cash
2. Revenue
3. Expense
4. Capital

82. A method of measuring the potential profitability of an investment, calculated by dividing the net income by the investment, is the _____. (*p. 289*)
1. Activity-based costing
2. ARR (accounting rate of return)
3. Profit ratio
4. Profit assurance calculation

83. A revision of an accounting forecast or assumption about the facility's expected or experienced performance is a(an) _____. (*p. 289*)
1. Change in accounting estimate
2. Change in performance
3. Review
4. Accountant's revision

84. The portion of a brand in the form of a symbol, design, or distinctive coloring or lettering, also called a logo, is an organization's _____. (*p. 290*)
   1. Intangible asset
   2. Sign
   3. Brand mark
   4. Original art

85. The administrator decides to offer newer forms of physical therapy that reduce use of currently used physical therapy methods. The administrator has _____ the current methods. (*p. 291*)
   1. Reduced the competitive advantage of
   2. Cannibalized
   3. Reduced
   4. Usurped

86. A market that is so competitive that all its participants have virtually no control over price is known as _____. (*p. 292*)
   1. Niche marketing
   2. No holds barred competition
   3. Perfect competition
   4. Imperfect markets

87. The administrator asks the business manager to divide the net income after any taxes by the noncurrent liabilities plus owners' equity. The administrator wants the _____. (*p. 293*)
   1. Best income estimate
   2. Return on invested capital estimate
   3. Probability estimate
   4. Best productivity achievable

88. A method of determining the optimum amount of materials that needs to be ordered on a regular basis is known as the _____. (*p. 296*)
   1. Best ordering method
   2. Ordering queue
   3. Economic order quantity
   4. Inventory control procedure

89. When governments use their powers to keep the price either above or below the equilibrium point it is known as _____. (*p. 297*)
   1. Market interference
   2. Government control
   3. Price controls
   4. Government rule

90. Short-term securities (2 days to 270 days) issued by corporations, banks, and other borrowing institutions to raise short-term working capital is known as _____. (p. 297)
    1. Securities fraud
    2. Commercial paper
    3. Short-term bonds
    4. Notes payable

91. The administrator asks the bank for an instrument stating that the bank that has granted the holder the amount of credit equal to the face amount wants a _____. (p. 297)
    1. Short-term loan
    2. Long-term loan
    3. Letter of credit
    4. Letter of assurance

92. The facility has issued a debt obligation to pay a specific amount on a stated date. The facility has issued _____. (p. 298)
    1. Letters of credit
    2. Notes
    3. Bonds
    4. Financial instruments

93. When the financial manager classifies an expense as an asset because it benefits the facility for more than 1 year, the financial manager has _____ that expense. (p. 298)
    1. Adjusted
    2. Reduced
    3. Spread
    4. Capitalized

94. The administrator wishes to lease a building and acquire substantial property rights in the process. The administrator seeks _____. (p. 298)
    1. A leasehold
    2. A long-term lease
    3. A capital lease
    4. Refinancing

95. The administrator has borrowed cash for an agreed upon purpose between a lender and borrower. The administrator now has a _____. (p. 299)
    1. Legal obligation
    2. Bond
    3. Note
    4. Capital asset

96. The chain issues stocks and bonds that can be converted into capital stock at some future date. It has issued _____. (*p. 299*)
    1. Convertible bonds
    2. Convertible securities
    3. Quasi-bonds
    4. Quasi-bonds and quasi-stocks

97. The chain "buys back" a portion of its outstanding stock by giving one new share in place of each four previously held shares. The chain has accomplished a(an) _____. (*p. 300*)
    1. Reverse split
    2. Buy-back
    3. Buy-down
    4. Illegal move

98. The administrator seeks to be licensed without having to meet all the conditions new entrants would have to meet. The administrator seeks to be _____. (*p. 300*)
    1. Grandfathered
    2. Granted concessions
    3. Avoiding current requirements
    4. Advancing him- or herself

99. The administrator holds a number of assets, such as bonds or easily sold stock, as investments. The administrator has substantial _____. (*p. 301*)
    1. Sources of income
    2. Riches
    3. Good investments
    4. Cash equivalents

100. The instrument that creates a corporation under the laws of a state is known as the _____. (*p. 302*)
    1. Registration
    2. Certificate
    3. Statement of incorporation
    4. Articles of incorporation

101. The three owners hold all the shares in the facility. They have a _____. (*p. 304*)
    1. Cash cow
    2. Profitable operation
    3. Semipublic corporation
    4. Privately held company

3.10.1 SOURCES OF LAW and
3.10.2 THE COURT SYSTEMS

1. Statutes are laws _____. (*p. 274*)
   1. Known as common law
   2. Made by judges
   3. Passed by cities
   4. Passed by legislatures

2. Normally, courts of appeal do not have _____. (*p. 276*)
   1. Criminal jurisdiction
   2. Original jurisdiction
   3. Criminal law enforcement authority
   4. Authority to hear misdemeanors

3. Statutes and subsequent regulations are collected in _____. (*p. 275*)
   1. The Code
   2. Constitutional amendments
   3. The federal requirements
   4. Law books

4. Generally, the lowest level of the court system is the _____ court. (*p. 275*)
   1. Circuit
   2. Criminal
   3. Civil
   4. Magistrate's

3.10.3 LEGAL TERMINOLOGY

5. To set a person or corporation free of accusations is to _____. (*p. 276*)
   1. Enjoin
   2. Acquit
   3. Consent
   4. Motion

6. A statement in writing given under oath before a notary public is an _____. (*p. 276*)
   1. Affidavit
   2. Affirmation
   3. Appeal
   4. Appearance

7. The coming into court of a person being summoned to do so is a(an) _____.
   (p. 277)
   1. Appeal
   2. Discovery
   3. Appearance
   4. Injunction

8. An impartial person chosen by the parties to an argument who agree to abide
   by that person's decision is a(an) _____. (p. 277)
   1. Arbitrator
   2. Adjudicator
   3. Civil judge
   4. Attorney at law

9. A Latin phrase meaning to stand by earlier court decisions is _____. (p. 279)
   1. Stare decisis
   2. Res judicata
   3. Res ipsa loquitur
   4. Respondeat superior

10. A verdict given by a jury at the direction of a judge is a(an) _____. (p. 278)
    1. Directed verdict
    2. Dismissal
    3. Indictment
    4. Injunction

11. An application to the court asking for an action favorable to one's side is _____.
    (p. 279)
    1. A witnessing
    2. A motion
    3. An application to the court
    4. A plea bargain

12. When the employee is acting within the control or scope of the employer, the
    employer is responsible for the acts of the employee under the concept of _____.
    (p. 282)
    1. Contractor–employee relations
    2. Strict liability
    3. A subcontractor relationship
    4. Borrowed servant

13. A written publication that exposes someone to public scorn, hatred, contempt,
    or ridicule is _____. (p. 278)
    1. Libel
    2. Slander
    3. An aggrieved party
    4. An assault

14. An early step in a criminal procedure during which the defendant is formally charged with an offense is a(an) _____. (*p. 277*)
    1. Discovery
    2. Arraignment
    3. Adjudication
    4. Action

15. Conduct giving rise to a cause for legal action is _____. (*p. 276*)
    1. Actionable
    2. An adjudication
    3. An appeal
    4. An indictment

16. When parties to a lawsuit who are dissatisfied with the court's decision ask a higher court to review the decision, it is known as a(an) _____. (*p. 276*)
    1. Appeal
    2. Arbitration
    3. Respondeat superior
    4. Stare decisis

17. A district attorney may bring assault charges for the purpose of _____. (*p. 280*)
    1. Revenge
    2. Punishment
    3. Monetary award
    4. Defamation

18. Damages for proven losses are known as _____ damages. (*p. 277*)
    1. Actual
    2. Exemplary
    3. Incidental
    4. Punitive

19. A fee paid in advance to an attorney for services on a case is known as a _____. (*p. 280*)
    1. Lien
    2. Prepayment
    3. Retainer
    4. Reward

20. A concept in torts used as a defense by the defendant against the plaintiff is an assumption of _____. (*p. 278*)
    1. The risk
    2. Innocence
    3. Guilt
    4. Fraud

21. Consent given after full information regarding the matter has been provided is known as _____ consent. (*p. 277*)
    1. Informed
    2. Individual
    3. Intended
    4. Personal

22. Spoken statements leading to actual damages implying crime, or unchastity, or relating to a person's profession or business are known as _____. (*p. 278*)
    1. Libel
    2. Slander
    3. Exemplary damages
    4. Consequential damages

23. A reckless disregard for human life, a state of mind that accompanies a wrongful act in which the resulting harm was intended, is known as _____. (*p. 278*)
    1. Malice
    2. Comparative negligence
    3. A heinous act
    4. Contempt

24. A public official, either elected or appointed, who conducts cases against persons accused of crimes is known as a _____. (*p. 279*)
    1. Lawyer
    2. Prosecutor
    3. Judge
    4. Bailiff

25. A written order from a judge permitting certain law enforcement officers to look for certain things or persons is a _____. (*p. 280*)
    1. Retainer
    2. Search certificate
    3. Search and rescue
    4. Search warrant

26. A person who gives evidence before a court and swears that testimony is true is a _____. (*p. 281*)
    1. Clerk of court
    2. Bailiff
    3. Sheriff
    4. Witness

27. A _____ exists when a legal duty is owed another, that duty is breached, and harm results. (*p. 280*)
    1. Tort
    2. Lien
    3. Deposition
    4. Warrant

28. A written order from a judge having authority in that jurisdiction for the arrest of a person is known as a _____. (*p. 281*)
    1. Tort
    2. Summons
    3. Warrant
    4. Directed verdict

3.10.4 RISKS ASSUMED BY THE OPERATION OF A LONG-TERM CARE FACILITY

29. The concept, in both civil and criminal law, that the employer is responsible without the employee having to show employer fault, and that normally applies to an ultra-hazardous situation is _____. (*p. 282*)
    1. Scope of employment
    2. Respondeat superior
    3. Contractor
    4. Strict liability

30. The range of employee activities held by the courts to be the legal responsibility of the employer, essentially any act performed in the process of carrying out one's duties, is known as _____. (*p. 282*)
    1. Scope of employment
    2. Range of job activities
    3. Employee job assignments
    4. Zone of employment

31. Laws that generally establish employer responsibility without regard to fault or negligence for employees' illnesses or injuries that arise out of performance of the job are known as _____. (*p. 282*)
    1. Worker's Compensation Act
    2. Employer's Liability Act
    3. Worker Insurance Program
    4. Worker Protection Act

32. Statutes in various states setting forth the extent to which employers are liable in regard to their employees are _____. (*p. 282*)
    1. Employer's Liability Acts
    2. Borrowed Servant Acts
    3. Contractor Acts
    4. Employee's Rights Laws

33. Under the concept of respondeat superior, the administration of the facility is as _____ responsible for the acts of contracted services as for acts of full-time employees. (*p. 282*)
   1. Partially
   2. Legally
   3. All too often
   4. Too infrequently

34. It normally falls to the _____ to ensure that contracted services are coordinated and supervised on an ongoing basis. (*p. 295*)
   1. Business office
   2. Corporate office
   3. Regional administrator
   4. Administrator

NAB Domain: Environment

Learning the Continuum of Long-Term Care

4.1 ORIGINS, OVERVIEW, AND CURRENT PROFILE OF THE NURSING HOME INDUSTRY

1. During the years 1993 to 2006, the percentage of chain-owned nursing facilities _____. (*p. 321*)*
   1. Was about 5%
   2. Varied between just less than and just more than half
   3. Doubled
   4. Tripled

2. During the years 1993 to 2006, the occupancy rates for U.S. nursing facilities _____. (*p. 322*)
   1. Remained unchanged
   2. Decreased
   3. Continued to increase slightly
   4. Increased as hospital discharge rates spiked

3. As a result of few new nursing homes being built in recent decades, it can be expected that occupancy rates in nursing homes _____ over the next 30 years. (*pp. 322–323*)
   1. Will remain level
   2. Will decrease
   3. May decrease
   4. Will be near 100%

---

*Answers can be found in *Nursing Home Administration*, Seventh Edition, on the page numbers in parentheses following each question.

4. The projections of daily volume of long-term care assistance by all categories of caregivers are expected to _____. (*p. 320*)
   1. Increase marginally
   2. Steadily increase
   3. Decrease as older persons get healthier
   4. Decrease

5. The projections of daily volume of long-term care assistance needed in the year 2040 are about _____ the need identified in 1980. (*p. 320*)
   1. Equal to
   2. Twice
   3. Three times
   4. Four times

6. The percentage of Medicaid dollars spent on institutional care over the past couple of decades has _____. (*p. 317*)
   1. Increased dramatically
   2. Decreased slightly
   3. Been unchanged
   4. Doubled

7. The American Association of Homes and Services for the Aging is the _____. (*p. 340*)
   1. National for-profit group
   2. National non-for-profit group
   3. Federal regional authority
   4. National federal authority

8. The proportion of Medicare nursing home residents who reside in facilities at any one time is _____ the proportion who are Medicaid.
   1. About equal to
   2. Far smaller than
   3. Far larger than
   4. Larger and growing

4.2 THE SOCIAL SECURITY ACT: MEDICARE AND MEDICAID

1. The federal government matches state expenditures ranging from _____. (*p. 343*)
   1. 50% to 83%
   2. 50% to 95%
   3. 40% to 60%
   4. 25% to 45%

2. In 2006, the federal government changed the "look back" period for which Medicaid assistance may be denied due to "gifts" _____. (*p. 349*)
   1. To cover only the medically indigent
   2. To relax the rules
   3. To provide relief to middle-class elderly
   4. From 3 years to 5 years look back

4.5 WORKPLACE SAFETY: THE OCCUPATIONAL SAFETY AND HEALTH ACT

3. Knowing the Occupational Safety and Health Act (OSHA) standards applicable to a facility is the responsibility of the _____. (*p. 379*)
   1. OSHA board
   2. Employer (the administrator)
   3. State Enforcement Commission
   4. Staff

4. Occupational Safety and Health Act (OSHA) inspectors examine the records of illnesses and injuries to the _____. (*p. 379*)
   1. Residents
   2. Employees
   3. Supervisors
   4. Residents and the employees

5. Accidents and illnesses requiring first aid and not resulting in work loss _____ reported. (*p. 380*)
   1. Do not have to be
   2. Must be
   3. Should be
   4. Must always be

4.6 FIRE SAFETY: THE LIFE SAFETY CODE®

6. The *Life Safety Code®* _____. (*p. 383*)
   1. Is too often ignored by states
   2. Must be used in every state
   3. Is fully voluntary for cities and counties
   4. Has the effect of law in most states

7. An employee hearing the fire code phrase must _____. (*p. 386*)
   1. Exit the facility
   2. Help fellow employees as needed
   3. Go to his or her assigned station
   4. Ask nearby persons where the fire is located

8. Under the *Life Safety Code®*, movement of infirm patients to safe areas or the exterior is _____ in fire drills. (*p. 385*)
   1. Required
   2. Not required
   3. At the option of the local fire chief
   4. Optional

9. On discovery of fire involving a person, personnel shall immediately _____. (*p. 386*)
   1. Assist the person
   2. Transmit a fire alarm
   3. Aid the person and call aloud "fire"
   4. Aid the person while calling aloud an established code phrase

10. Basic action required of health care facility personnel is _____. (*p. 385*)
    1. Removal of directly involved occupants
    2. Transmission of an alarm signal
    3. Confinement of the effects of the fire
    4. All of the aforementioned

11. Often the most dangerous element threatening patient safety is _____. (*p. 387*)
    1. Unavailability of correct type of extinguisher
    2. Slow-thinking responses by personnel
    3. Smoke inhalation
    4. First- and second-degree burns

12. Smoking by residents designated as "not responsible" _____. (*p. 386*)
    1. Is permitted for the terminally ill
    2. Must be closely supervised
    3. Is prohibited
    4. Must be in a safe area

13. The overall objective of the *Life Safety Code®* for new health care occupancies is to _____. (*p. 385*)
    1. Limit spread of a fire to the room of fire origin
    2. Require sprinkler systems or their equivalent as applicable
    3. Educate the public on correct fire procedures
    4. Provide guidelines for the local fire chief

14. Facility personnel who shall be instructed in the use of and response to a fire alarm include _____. (*p. 386*)
    1. Nursing staff
    2. All staff having patient contact
    3. Nursing and dietary staff
    4. All personnel

15. When a facility locks exits, it must _____. (*p. 386*)
    1. Hire additional staff
    2. Use special locks
    3. Get permission from the local fire marshal
    4. Maintain adequate staff to release locks

16. A material that, in the form in which it is used, will not aid combustion or add appreciable heat to spreading fire is defined as _____. (*p. 386*)
    1. Fire resistant
    2. Fire coded
    3. Noncombustible
    4. Combustible

17. In determining occupant loads in exit requirements, the actual expected count or a projection using _____ square feet of floor space in sleeping areas and _____ square feet of floor space in treatment areas shall be used. (*p. 390*)
    1. 120/240
    2. 100/200
    3. 220/440
    4. 440/640

18. Handrails clearance from the wall must be at least _____. (*p. 390*)
    1. 1 hand wide
    2. 6 inches
    3. 1 and one-half inches
    4. 8 inches

19. The purpose of smoke-proof towers is to _____. (*p. 390*)
    1. Limit infiltration of heat, smoke, and fire gases
    2. Contain construction costs
    3. Improve the visual appeal of the building
    4. Totally eliminate smoke and gases

20. The National Safety Council has suggested slopes of 7 to 20 degrees for a _____. (*p. 391*)
    1. Stairway
    2. Stairway and landings
    3. Stairway and ramp
    4. Ramp

21. Aisles, corridors, and ramps used for exit must be at least _____ in width, and clear and unobstructed. (*p. 391*)
    1. 8 feet
    2. 3 feet
    3. Within residents' ability to move
    4. Reasonably wide

22. Travel distance within a room to an exit must not exceed _____. (*p. 391*)
    1. 25 yards
    2. 50 feet
    3. Good judgment
    4. Local fire marshal rules

23. Each floor or fire section of the facility shall have at least _____ located _____ from each other. (*p. 391*)
    1. Three exits/remotely
    2. Two exits/remotely
    3. Two ramps/away
    4. Three ramps/remotely

24. Travel distance from within any patient room to an exit access must not exceed _____. (*p. 391*)
    1. 50 feet
    2. 75 feet
    3. 100 feet
    4. 200 feet

25. Illumination of the means of egress must be continuous and must provide at least _____ foot-candle(s) measured at the _____. (*p. 391*)
    1. 1/floor
    2. 2/railings
    3. 1/railing
    4. 2/floor

26. The emergency lighting system must provide power _____. (*p. 391*)
    1. Automatically
    2. With a minimum of operations
    3. From each nursing station
    4. From a switch in the administrator's office

27. Exit signs must be placed so that a person is never more than _____ from the nearest exit sign. (*p. 392*)
    1. 50 feet
    2. 100 feet
    3. 150 feet
    4. 200 feet

28. Corridors throughout patient sleeping areas must have _____. (*p. 393*)
    1. Automatic smoke detection systems
    2. 9 feet in clearance
    3. Well-decorated walls
    4. Smooth surfaces

29. A supervised automatic sprinkler system _____. (p. 393)
    1. Is advised
    2. Should be installed
    3. Is a luxury for the average nursing facility
    4. Is required

30. Short persons must be able to reach _____. (p. 393)
    1. Fire extinguishers
    2. Door stops
    3. Top shelves
    4. Top of bureaus

31. A fixed, regularly serviced, automatic fire extinguishing system in nursing home kitchens over the cook stoves is _____. (p. 392)
    1. Required
    2. Permitted in most states
    3. Highly recommended
    4. Optional

32. Every building shall have a(an) _____ operated fire alarm system that shall be _____ supervised. (p. 393)
    1. Sprinkler/continuously
    2. Automatic/continuously
    3. Simultaneously/continuously
    4. Manually/electronically

33. Every story used by patients must be divided into _____. (p. 394)
    1. Four smoke compartments
    2. Equal spaces
    3. Two smoke compartments
    4. Five smoke compartments

34. Every story with 50 or more occupants must be divided into at least _____. (p. 394)
    1. Six rooms
    2. Two smoke compartments
    3. Two nursing stations responsibilities
    4. Four smoke compartments

35. Extinguishers should be checked _____ by the fire department and recharged and serviced _____ by a qualified person. (p. 393)
    1. Monthly/monthly
    2. Monthly/quarterly
    3. Monthly/annually
    4. Quarterly/annually

36. Doors protecting corridor openings must be made of 1¾ inches solid bonded core wood or constructed to resist fire for at least _____ minutes. (*p. 394*)
    1. 10
    2. 20
    3. 60
    4. 45

37. Each patient room must have an outside window or door. If a window, it _____.
    (*p. 394*)
    1. Must be at least 2 feet by 4 feet
    2. Must have a latch on it
    3. Need not be operable
    4. Must be Thermopane

4.7 AMERICANS WITH DISABILITIES ACT (ADA) ACCESSIBILITY GUIDELINES FOR FACILITIES

38. For changes in level: up to ¼ inch _____, between ¼ and ½ inch _____ is required, and more than ½ inch must meet _____ requirements. (*p. 400*)
    1. Permissible/beveled edge/ramp
    2. Ignored/curved edge/grade
    3. Permitted/sharp edge/ramp
    4. Required/rounded edge/grade

39. On any given flight of stairs, riser heights and tread widths must be _____.
    (*p. 403*)
    1. Uniform
    2. Appropriate
    3. Approved
    4. Cleared with the architect

40. High forward reach limit is generally _____. (*p. 399*)
    1. 5 feet
    2. 6 feet
    3. 48 inches
    4. Up to the facility to determine

41. Minimum width for two wheelchairs to pass is _____ inches. (*p. 399*)
    1. 40
    2. 60
    3. 72
    4. 82

42. Side reach should be between _____ inches off the floor. (*p. 399*)
    1. 9 and 54
    2. 20 and 40
    3. 60 and 70
    4. 12 and 24

43. Handrails must extend at least _____ inches beyond a ramp or stair and be parallel to the floor or ground surface. (*p. 408*)
    1. 4
    2. 6
    3. 8
    4. 12

44. The generally specified maximum pounds of pressure required to operate doors, windows, and so on, is _____. (*p. 409*)
    1. 1
    2. 3
    3. 5
    4. 10

45. Automatic doors and power-assisted doors should be slow opening and low powered, not opening back to back faster than _____ seconds nor with a force of more than _____ pounds. (*p. 409*)
    1. 3/15
    2. 5/20
    3. 10/30
    4. 15/45

46. Grab bars located between _____ and _____ inches high must be provided for toilets on the side and back walls. (*p. 411*)
    1. 33/36
    2. 30/40
    3. 20/40
    4. 25/45

47. Grab bars and handrails are to be _____ to _____ inches in diameter or width, with _____ inches space between handrail and wall, and a sheer stress point of _____ pounds or greater. (*pp. 414–415*)
    1. 1/2/2/200
    2. 1¼/1½/1½/250
    3. 2/4/6/500
    4. 4/4/6/600

48. The maximum allowable emergency alarm level is _____ decibels. (*p. 415*)
1. 60
2. 80
3. 100
4. 120

49. The general requirement for knee clearance under tables, work surfaces, sinks, and lavatories is _____. (*p. 417*)
1. 10 inches
2. 19 inches
3. 1 foot
4. 2 feet

50. Title 7 of the Civil Rights Act of 1964 prohibited employers from discriminating on the basis of _____. (*p. 160*)
1. All of the following
2. Race
3. Color
4. Sex

51. In 1935, a major labor group emerged called the _____. (*p. 358*)
1. CIO (Congress of Industrial Organizations)
2. AFL (American Federation of Labor)
3. AFL-CIO
4. National Unions Group

52. By 1947, unions represented about 31% of the workforce. In 2015, union membership represented about ____% of the total work force. (*p. 362*)
1. 11
2. 16
3. 30
4. 40

53. The Taft-Hartley Act prohibited managers from _____. (*p. 359*)
1. Giving tenure to employees to discourage unionization
2. Giving wage increases to discourage unionization
3. Firing employees who give testimony under the Wagner Act
4. All of the aforementioned

54. The National Labor Relations Board (NLRB) does not _____. (*p. 360*)
1. Determine what the bargaining units shall be
2. Conduct representative elections by secret ballot
3. Investigate unfair labor practices
4. Make court decisions

55. In 1973, the hospitals and nursing facility interests did not seek _____. (*p. 361*)
    1. Exemption from National Labor Relations Board (NLRB) oversight
    2. Priority for National Labor Relations Board (NLRB) actions on disputes
    3. Mandatory mediation requirements
    4. Limit on number of bargaining units

56. In 1984, the National Labor Relations Board (NLRB) favored nursing home managers by ruling that the appropriate bargaining unit is _____. (*p. 361*)
    1. All professionals, all nonprofessionals
    2. Some professionals, all nonprofessionals
    3. Most professionals, most nonprofessionals
    4. Workers, managers

57. Discrimination was interpreted initially by the courts as harmful action, later as unequal treatment, and more recently as _____. (*p. 363*)
    1. Unequal or adverse impact
    2. Unjustifiable
    3. Rule of the 1980s
    4. Wrongdoing

58. The Civil Rights Act is enforced _____. (*p. 365*)
    1. By the Equal Opportunities Commission
    2. By the Equal Employment Commission
    3. By the Equal Employment Opportunity Commission
    4. Solely by the federal courts

59. The Fair Labor Standards Act requires that an overtime rate of _____ times the hourly (or other basis) rates be paid for all hours more than _____ during the week. (*p. 373*)
    1. 2/40
    2. 1½/40
    3. 2/35
    4. 2/45

60. Minors younger than 16 years may not be employed in the nursing facility except under _____. (*p. 374*)
    1. Temporary conditions
    2. Parental consent (must be written)
    3. Situations of clear need
    4. A temporary permit issued by the Department of Labor

61. Funds for unemployment compensation come from a _____ payroll tax based on wages of each employee up to a certain _____. (*p. 376*)
    1. State/minimum
    2. Federal/minimum
    3. Federal/maximum
    4. Local/maximum

62. Under ERISA (Employee Retirement Income Security Act of 1975), employers _____ pension plan. (*p. 376*)
    1. Are required to offer a
    2. Are not required to offer a
    3. Must enlarge their existing
    4. Are prohibited from offering a

4.8 EXPANDING FACILITY SERVICES: HEALTH PLANNING REGULATIONS

63. In states where a local health planning agency believes a shortage of nursing home beds exists, it may _____. (*p. 420*)
    1. Require additional beds be built
    2. Let a contract for building new beds
    3. Advertise for beds
    4. Issue a certificate of need

64. The most well-known model of the grieving process was developed by an American psychiatrist _____ in the book, *On Death and Dying*. (*p. 331*)
    1. Elizabeth Taylor
    2. Elisabeth Kübler-Ross
    3. Freud
    4. Jung

65. The five stages of dying are thought to be denial, anger, bargaining, depression, and _____. (*p. 331*)
    1. Death
    2. Acceptance
    3. Final denial
    4. Futility

66. Basically, under the Privacy Rule issued by the Department of Health and Human Services (DHHS), it is illegal for any person to gain access to personal medical information for any reason other than health care delivery, operations, and _____. (*p. 371*)
    1. Supplemental income
    2. Charging
    3. Reimbursement
    4. Refunds

67. The following are _____:

- Hepatitis B
- Influenza
- Measles
- Mumps
- Rubella
- Varicella
- Tetanus
- Diphtheria
- Pertussis. (*p. 382*)

1. Recommended vaccines for health care workers
2. Required patient vaccines
3. Suggested mass inoculations
4. Nursing personnel vaccines

68. The _____ required insurance companies to cover all applicants within new minimum standards and offer the same rates regardless of preexisting conditions or sex. (*p. 423*)
1. Health Care Act
2. Universal Care Act
3. Affordable Care Act
4. Nursing Home Care Program

69. The _____ includes a requirement that both the federal Department of Health and Human Services and local law enforcement authorities must be notified of any suspicions of abuse regardless of whether or not that suspected abuse results in bodily harm. (*p. 424*)
1. Health Care Act
2. Universal Care Act
3. Affordable Health Act
4. Elder Justice Law, 2010

4.9 VOLUNTARY OPERATING STANDARDS: THE JOINT COMMISSION ON ACCREDITATION OF HEALTH CARE ORGANIZATIONS

70. For nursing facilities, meeting requirements set by the Joint Commission on Accreditation of Healthcare Organizations (JCAHO) is _____. (*p. 422*)
1. Voluntary
2. Mandatory
3. Required for Medicaid payments
4. Required for Medicare payments

NAB Domain: Patient/Resident Care

Building Your Resident Care Skills

5.1 THE AGING PROCESS: OVERVIEW AND THEORIES

1. Which of the following is a safe generalization about aging? _____. (*p. 430*)*
   1. Old age ain't for sissies
   2. Aging is highly individualized
   3. Senility is inevitable
   4. Aging leads to dependency status

2. Professionals who study aging and are normally not physicians are called _____.
   (*p. 430*)
   1. Geriatricians
   2. Gerontologists
   3. Family practitioners
   4. Specialists

3. The progressive loss of cortical neurons (brain cells) and brain weight means that
   older persons _____. (*p. 431*)
   1. Begin to move more slowly
   2. Think less clearly
   3. Behave less predictably
   4. Are unaffected by the loss

4. Aging is a gradual decline of at least some of the systems in the body, which
   proceed _____. (*p. 431*)
   1. At different rates in different individuals
   2. At essentially the same rate for everyone
   3. At a rate unique to men and a rate unique to women
   4. Rapidly

---

*Answers can be found in *Nursing Home Administration*, Seventh Edition, on the page numbers in parentheses following each question.

5. According to Leonard Hayflick's theory, aging occurs because of _____ (*p. 433*)
   1. A limit of about 50 divisions for certain key groups of cells in humans
   2. Loss of collagen
   3. Wear and tear
   4. Progressive failure of the immune system

6. According to the autoimmune response theory of aging, "copying errors" in repeated cell divisions result in cells that are progressively not recognized by the body, leading to _____. (*p. 434*)
   1. Triggering the immune system to attack these cells
   2. Damage to the RNA
   3. Limited cell divisions
   4. Reduction in elasticity of vital body parts, such as the blood vessels

5.2 MEDICAL AND RELATED TERMS

5.2.1 SPECIALIZATIONS

1. Physicians who specialize in treating older persons are _____. (*p. 438*)
   1. Gerontologists
   2. Family doctors
   3. Geriatricians
   4. Specialists

2. A physician who diagnoses and treats diseases of the brain, nervous system, and spinal cord is a(an) _____. (*p. 438*)
   1. Ophthalmologist
   2. Optician
   3. Optometrist
   4. Neurologist

3. A technician, not a physician, trained to grind lenses and to fit them is a(an) _____. (*p. 438*)
   1. General surgeon
   2. Orthopedist
   3. Ophthalmologist
   4. Optician

4. A dentist who specializes in the extraction of teeth is a(an) _____.
   1. Osteopath
   2. Orthopedist
   3. Oral surgeon
   4. Periodontist

5. A physician who specializes in diagnostic procedures and treatment of nonsurgical cases is known as a(an) _____. (*p. 438*)
   1. Orthopedist
   2. Urologist
   3. Internist
   4. Externist

6. A physician who specializes in examination of body tissues under laboratory conditions is known as a(an) _____.
   1. Podiatrist
   2. Pathologist
   3. Internist
   4. Specialist

7. A physician who specializes in physical medicine, body movements, and conditioning is known as a _____. (*p. 438*)
   1. Pedodontist
   2. Pediatrician
   3. Physiatrist
   4. Podiatrist

8. A physician who specializes in the diagnosis and treatment of mental disorders is known as a(an) _____. (*p. 438*)
   1. Psychiatrist
   2. Psychologist
   3. Psychic advisor
   4. Exodontist

9. A physician specializing in the use of x-ray and similar medical diagnostic machines is known as a(an) _____. (*p. 438*)
   1. Radiologist
   2. Anesthesiologist
   3. Cardiologist
   4. Chiropractor

10. A psychiatrist who specializes in the use of psychoanalytic techniques of therapy is known as a(an) _____. (*p. 438*)
    1. Psychoanalyst
    2. Psychologist
    3. Pathologist
    4. Endocrinologist

11. A physician specializing in the diagnosis and treatment of the large intestine, particularly the rectum, is known as a(an) _____. (*p. 438*)
    1. Optometrist
    2. Podiatrist
    3. Proctologist
    4. Allergist

12. A physician specializing in treatment of the kidney and bladder is known as a(an) _____. (*p. 438*)
    1. Exodontist
    2. Urologist
    3. Periodontist
    4. Proctologist

13. A physician who specializes in the treatment of arthritic diseases is known as a(an) _____. (*p. 438*)
    1. Pedodontist
    2. Rheumatologist
    3. Orthodontist
    4. Orthopedist

14. A physician specializing in the treatment of the lungs is known as a(an) _____. (*p. 438*)
    1. Pulmonologist
    2. Periodontist
    3. Plastic surgeon
    4. Dental specialist

15. A physician who diagnoses and treats eye diseases and disorders, performs eye surgery, refracts the eyes, and prescribes corrective eyeglasses and lenses is known as a(an) _____. (*p. 438*)
    1. Optician
    2. Ophthalmologist
    3. Neurosurgeon
    4. Osteopath

5.2.2 MEDICATIONS/THERAPEUTIC ACTIONS OF DRUGS

1. Induces vomiting; for example, warm salt water: _____. (*p. 445*)
    1. Antiemetic
    2. Emetic
    3. Sedative
    4. Hypotensive drug

2. Destroys tissue by local application; for example, silver nitrate: _____. (*p. 445*)
    1. Caustic
    2. Mydriotic
    3. Carminative
    4. Diuretic

3. Expands or dilates blood vessels: _____. (*p. 445*)
   1. Vasodilators
   2. Vasoconstrictors
   3. Carminative
   4. Mydriatic

4. Reduces pain; for example, aspirin: _____. (*p. 445*)
   1. Analgesic
   2. Antiseptic
   3. Caustic
   4. Coagulant

5. Used in treatment of anemia; for example, liver extract _____. (*p. 445*)
   1. Antianemic
   2. Antispasmodic
   3. Hypnotic
   4. Diaphoretic

6. Helps raise blood pressure: _____. (*p. 445*)
   1. Vasodilator
   2. Hypotensive
   3. Hormone
   4. Hypertensive

7. Stimulates elimination of urine, often used with medications prescribed to reduce hypertension; for example, thiomirin: _____. (*p. 445*)
   1. Stimulant
   2. Expectorant
   3. Sedative
   4. Diuretic

8. Slows down growth of bacteria, but does not kill all of the bacteria; for example, hydrogen peroxide: _____. (*p. 445*)
   1. Antacid
   2. Antitoxin
   3. Antiseptic
   4. Astringent

9. Used to induce coughing; an agent that increases bronchial secretion and facilitates its expulsion; for example, Robitussin: _____. (*p. 445*)
   1. Expectorant
   2. Emollient
   3. Cathartic
   4. Carminative

10. Destroys microorganisms in the body; for example, penicillin: _____. (*p. 445*)
    1. Antacids
    2. Mydriotic
    3. Emollient
    4. Antibiotic

11. Laxatives, purgatives, inducing bowel movements; for example, cascara sagrada: _____. (*p. 445*)
    1. Antacid
    2. Cathartic
    3. Antispasmodic
    4. Hypotensive

12. Destroys pathogenic organism; for example, zepharin chloride: _____. (*p. 445*)
    1. Diaphoretic
    2. Antibiotic
    3. Antitoxin
    4. Disinfectant

13. Used to induce perspiration: _____. (*p. 445*)
    1. Emollient
    2. Miotic
    3. Diaphoretic
    4. Mydriatic

14. Relieves smooth muscle contraction; for example, diazepam (Valium): _____. (*p. 445*)
    1. Antianemic
    2. Anticoagulant
    3. Antidote
    4. Antispasmodic

15. Causes the blood vessels to narrow or constrict: _____. (*p. 445*)
    1. Vasodilator
    2. Vasoconstrictor
    3. Antispasmodic
    4. Antacid

16. Decreases clotting of the blood: _____. (*p. 445*)
    1. Antitoxin
    2. Anticoagulant
    3. Antianemic
    4. Coagulant

5.2.3 ABBREVIATIONS

1. diag. (*p. 446*)
1. Diagnosis
2. Diagram
3. Down from
4. Diagrammatic

2. BMR (*p. 446*)
1. Basic medicinal regimen
2. Basal metabolic rate
3. Base mass required
4. None of these is correct

3. noct. (*p. 447*)
1. Notch
2. At night
3. Nosocomial
4. Notice

4. W/C (*p. 448*)
1. Whooping cough
2. Whiplash characteristic
3. Whip chalasia
4. Wheelchair

5. stat. (*p. 448*)
1. Stationary
2. Statistic
3. Sustained
4. Immediately

6. URI (*p. 448*)
1. Upper respiratory infection
2. Upper resting indicator
3. Upper resistance indicator
4. Upper reading indicated

7. Omn. hor.
1. Every 10 hours
2. Every day
3. Every hour
4. Each night

8. gm. (*p. 447*)
  1. Gamma globule
  2. Grand mal (epilepsy)
  3. Groin
  4. Gram

9. cf. (*p. 446*)
  1. Compare
  2. Confused
  3. Confrontational
  4. Amount

10. NPO (*p. 447*)
  1. Nothing by mouth
  2. Nothing postoperative
  3. Note after (the) operation
  4. Noted by operator

11. Ad. lib. (*p. 446*)
  1. As much as desired
  2. Toward the left
  3. Administrative liberty
  4. Alternate days

12. exam. (*p. 446*)
  1. Example
  2. Exaggerated
  3. Examination
  4. Review

13. RBC
  1. Resting blood count
  2. Red blood count
  3. Retinal blastoma corion
  4. None of these is correct

14. TO (*p. 448*)
  1. Per operator
  2. By mouth
  3. Telephone order
  4. Per observations

15. Rx. (*p. 448*)
  1. Rexall
  2. Prescription
  3. Relaxation
  4. Rectally

16. spec. (*p. 448*)
1. Special
2. Specific
3. Speculation
4. Specimen

17. ung. (*p. 448*)
1. Ointment
2. Ungrateful
3. Unguinal
4. Ungulate

18. VO (*p. 448*)
1. Volume observed
2. Velocity observation
3. Verbal order
4. Vital observation

19. BE (*p. 446*)
1. Barium enema
2. Best estimate
3. Most efficient
4. Bronchial emphysema

20. PRN (*p. 447*)
1. As directed
2. As ordered
3. As needed
4. As observed

21. tab. (*p. 448*)
1. (To) tabulate
2. Tablet
3. Total
4. Tabescent

22. Disch. (*p. 446*)
1. Discharge
2. Discontinue
3. Disengage
4. Disease

23. Omn. noct.
1. All requirements
2. Omentum
3. Omentitis
4. Every night

24. tid (*p. 448*)
1. Treble in dosage
2. Three times a day
3. Triple in dosage
4. Trigonitis

25. qd (*p. 447*)
1. Hourly
2. Weekly
3. Daily
4. Quotient

26. IV (*p. 447*)
1. Intravenous
2. Intravital
3. Intraventricular
4. Intravasion

27. h.s. (*p. 447*)
1. Hospital
2. At bedtime
3. On rising
4. Hyaloserositis

28. inf. (*p. 447*)
1. Infinity
2. Infantilism
3. Infusion
4. Infiltration

29. FUO (*p. 447*)
1. Fracture of unknown origin
2. Fistula of unknown origin
3. Fever of unknown origin
4. Fibrosis of unknown origin

30. EEG (*p. 446*)
1. Electroencephalogram
2. Electrocardiogram
3. Exciting electrode graphics
4. Electrogastrograph

31. sol. (*p. 448*)
1. Solution
2. Solar
3. Sole
4. Sun

32. u. (*p. 448*)
1. Unfit
2. Undo
3. Urgent
4. Unit

33. surg. (*p. 448*)
1. Surrogate
2. Surgery
3. Surgical
4. Susceptible

34. lab. (*p. 447*)
1. Labiograph
2. Labionasal
3. Laboratory
4. Labiogingival

5.2.4 PREFIXES

1. a-, an-; for example, anorexia: _____. (*p. 448*)
1. Without
2. Down from
3. Away from
4. Decreasing

2. ad-; for example, additive: _____. (*p. 448*)
1. Toward, to, at
2. From
3. Away
4. Decreasing

3. ambi-; for example, ambilateral: _____. (*p. 449*)
1. Additional
2. Reducing
3. Confusing
4. Both

4. angio-; for example, angiofibrosis: _____. (*p. 449*)
1. Relating to
2. To a vessel
3. Against
4. Differentiated from

5. antero-; for example, anteromedian _____. (*p. 449*)
   1. In front of
   2. Away from
   3. Down from
   4. Relating to

6. apo-; for example, apocleisis: _____.
   1. Relating to
   2. Many
   3. Up, toward
   4. Away from, off

7. arthro-; for example, arthropathy: _____. (*p. 449*)
   1. Relation to the legs
   2. Relation to the joints
   3. Relation to the neck
   4. Relation to an arthritic condition

8. bi-; for example, bilateral: _____. (*p. 449*)
   1. Together
   2. Pertaining to
   3. Good
   4. Two

9. brady-; for example, bradycardia: _____. (*p. 449*)
   1. Fast
   2. Slow
   3. On the side of
   4. Head

10. carcino-; for example, carcinogen: _____. (*p. 449*)
    1. Pertaining to additives
    2. Pertaining to poisons
    3. Pertaining to a reduction
    4. Pertaining to cancer

11. cata-; for example, catabolism: _____. (*p. 449*)
    1. Toward
    2. Downward, against
    3. Deriving from
    4. Within, inner

12. cephalo-; for example, cephalogram: _____. (*p. 449*)
    1. Neck
    2. Shoulder
    3. Trunk of body
    4. Head

13. chiro-; for example, chiroplasty: _____. (*p. 449*)
    1. Pertaining to the hand
    2. Pertaining to the neck
    3. Pertaining to the body
    4. Pertaining to the head

14. circum-; for example, circumcorneal: _____. (*p. 449*)
    1. Under
    2. Beneath
    3. Above
    4. Around

15. contra-; for example, contraindicated: _____. (*p. 449*)
    1. Without
    2. Around
    3. Above
    4. Against, opposite

16. cranio-; for example, craniotomy: _____. (*p. 450*)
    1. Pertaining to the neck
    2. Pertaining to the spinal cord
    3. Pertaining to the head
    4. Pertaining to the lower back

17. cyto-; for example, cytolysis: _____. (*p. 450*)
    1. Relation to a cell
    2. Relation to life
    3. Relation to a limb
    4. A cleansing

18. derm-; for example, dermatitis: _____. (*p. 450*)
    1. Pertaining to the skin
    2. Pertaining to the lower intestine
    3. Relating to germs
    4. Pertaining to the skull

19. di-; for example, diarthric: _____. (*p. 450*)
    1. Through
    2. A cutting of
    3. Within
    4. Double, twice

20. dys-; for example, dysphasia: _____. (*p. 450*)
    1. Away from
    2. Down from
    3. Within
    4. Painful, difficult

21. em-, en-; for example, embolic: _____. (*p. 450*)
1. In
2. Outside of
3. Around
4. Through

22. endo-; for example, endocarditis: _____. (*p. 450*)
1. Within, inner
2. Exterior to
3. Pertaining to
4. Above

23. epi-; for example, epidermatitis: _____. (*p. 450*)
1. Above, upon, over
2. Below
3. Through
4. Surrounding

24. fibro-; for example, fibrocarcinoma: _____. (*p. 450*)
1. Pertaining to a large mass
2. Pertaining to fiber
3. Pertaining to a softening
4. Pertaining to diluting

25. glyco-; for example, glycosuria: _____. (*p. 450*)
1. Relation to sweetness
2. Relation to the head
3. A diminution or decrease
4. Relation to the stomach

26. hema-, hemo-; for example, hemorrhage: _____. (*p. 451*)
1. Pertaining to the liver
2. Pertaining to the pancreas
3. Pertaining to the ductless glands
4. Pertaining to the blood

27. hepato-; for example, hepatitis: _____. (*p. 451*)
1. Lung
2. Liver
3. Heart
4. Limb

28. hydro-; for example, hydrocyst: _____. (*p. 451*)
1. Lymph
2. Water
3. Bile
4. Any secretion

29. hypno-; for example, hypnotherapy: _____. (*p. 451*)
   1. Relating to water
   2. Relating to a drainage
   3. Relating to sleep
   4. Relating to depression

30. hystero-; for example, hysterogram: _____. (*p. 451*)
   1. Relating to the blood
   2. Relating to the cells
   3. Relating to the uterus
   4. A cutting out

31. infra-; for example, infracardiac: _____. (*p. 451*)
   1. Above
   2. Beneath, below
   3. Beside of
   4. In the direction of

32. intra-; for example, intracutaneous: _____.
   1. Within
   2. On the surface
   3. Exterior to
   4. Away from

33. osteo-; for example, osteoporosis: _____. (*p. 452*)
   1. Pertaining to an opening
   2. Pertaining to the bones
   3. Pertaining to the body
   4. Pertaining to the skull

34. pachy-; for example, pachylosis: _____. (*p. 452*)
   1. Thick
   2. Thin
   3. Scattered
   4. Uncoordinated

35. para-; for example, paralysis: _____.
   1. Between
   2. Beneath
   3. Instead of
   4. Beyond, beside

36. per-; for example, perfusion: _____. (*p. 452*)
   1. Through
   2. About
   3. Down from
   4. False

37. phlebo-; for example, phlebitis: _____. (*p. 452*)
   1. Relating to an artery
   2. Relating to phlegm
   3. Relating to a vein
   4. Relating to a nephron

38. poly-; for example, polycardia: _____. (*p. 452*)
   1. Many, much
   2. Happiness
   3. Depressed
   4. Shiny

39. pseudo-; for example, pseudodementia: _____. (*p. 452*)
   1. Many
   2. Fresh
   3. New
   4. False

40. pyo-; for example, pyoderma: _____. (*p. 452*)
   1. Signifying fire
   2. Signifying pus
   3. Signifying desire for a change
   4. Signifying a deepening

41. rhino-; for example, rhinoplasty: _____. (*p. 453*)
   1. A large beast
   2. Nose
   3. Liver
   4. Kidney

42. tachy-; for example, tachycardia: _____. (*p. 453*)
   1. Poor taste
   2. Rapid
   3. Slow
   4. Indifferent

43. uni-; for example, unicellular: _____. (*p. 453*)
   1. All
   2. Neither
   3. One
   4. Many

44. intro-; for example, introgastric: _____. (*p. 451*)
   1. In, into
   2. On the outside of
   3. Surrounding
   4. Below

45. labio-; for example, labiocervical: _____. (*p. 451*)
1. Relating to the lip
2. Relating to nearby tissues
3. Surrounding
4. Containing

46. mega-; for example, megacardia: _____. (*p. 451*)
1. Large, oversize
2. Relating to the intestines
3. Relating to the meninges
4. Relating to the brain

47. myo-; for example, myocardial infarction: _____. (*p. 452*)
1. Relating to an enlargement
2. Relating to a metastasis
3. Relating to muscle
4. Relating to nerve fibers

48. necro-; for example, necrosis: _____. (*p. 452*)
1. Darkening
2. Death
3. Enlargement
4. Shrinkage

49. omo-; for example, omodynia: _____. (*p. 452*)
1. Pertaining to the knee joint
2. Pertaining to the shoulder
3. A reduction
4. An unexplained enlargement

50. odont-; for example, odontalgia: _____. (*p. 452*)
1. Relating to the teeth
2. Relating to the upper back
3. Relating to the spine
4. Relating to an opening

5.2.5 SUFFIXES

1. -ac; for example, cardiac: _____. (*p. 452*)
1. Flowing from
2. Following
3. Pertaining to
4. Underneath

2. -algia; for example, neuralgia: _____. (*p. 453*)
   1. Heat
   2. A loss of
   3. Pleasure
   4. Pain

3. -centesis; for example, paracentesis: _____. (*p. 453*)
   1. Centered
   2. One-sided
   3. Occurring on both sides
   4. Surgical puncture

4. -clysis; for example, enteroclysis: _____. (*p. 453*)
   1. Controlling
   2. Reducing infection of
   3. Excision of
   4. Washing, irrigation

5. -cycle; for example, _____. (*pp. 453–454*)
   1. Organ
   2. Tissue
   3. Cell
   4. Appendage

6. -emesis; for example, hyperemesis: _____. (*p. 453*)
   1. Cleansing
   2. Vomiting
   3. Coughing
   4. Shrinking

7. -genesis; for example, carcinogenesis: _____. (*p. 453*)
   1. Condition of reducing
   2. Reshaping
   3. Reducing
   4. Condition of producing

8. -lith; for example, nephrolith: _____. (*p. 453*)
   1. Graph
   2. Chart
   3. Figure
   4. Stone

9. -malacia; for example, osteomalacia: _____. (*p. 453*)
   1. Hardening
   2. Softening
   3. Swelling
   4. Suture

10. -odynia; for example, cardiodynia: _____. (*p. 454*)
    1. A painful condition
    2. An improving condition
    3. A reduction in
    4. Reduction in size of

11. -opsy; for example, biopsy: _____. (*p. 454*)
    1. To view
    2. To reduce in size
    3. To excise
    4. To cut

12. -orrhaphy; for example, gastrorrhaphy: _____. (*p. 454*)
    1. Appetite, desire
    2. Deficiency
    3. To view
    4. Suture

13. -orrhea; for example, gastrorrhea: _____. (*p. 454*)
    1. Flow, discharge
    2. To view
    3. Incision
    4. Fixation

14. -otomy; for example, nephrotomy: _____. (*p. 454*)
    1. To remove
    2. Incision, to cut into
    3. A state of
    4. A poor prognosis

15. -penia; for example, leukopenia: _____. (*p. 454*)
    1. Excess
    2. Deficiency
    3. Discharge
    4. Tumor

16. -pexy; for example, nephropexy: _____. (*p. 454*)
    1. Disruption
    2. Discharge
    3. Seepage
    4. Fixation, to put into place

17. -phasia; for example, aphasia: _____.
    1. Spasm
    2. Hardening
    3. Softening
    4. Speech

18. -phobia; for example, claustrophobia: _____. (*p. 454*)
    1. Enjoyment
    2. Contentment
    3. Fear
    4. Speech

19. -rhythmia; for example, arrhythmia: _____. (*p. 454*)
    1. Rhythmic
    2. Rheumatoid
    3. Irregular
    4. Variegated

20. -spasm; for example, myospasm: _____. (*p. 454*)
    1. Sudden violent involuntary contraction of muscles
    2. Sudden violent voluntary contraction of muscles
    3. Outburst
    4. Hemorrhage

21. -stenosis; for example, arteriostenosis: _____.
    1. Widening
    2. Tightening, stricture
    3. Relaxation
    4. Spasm

22. -tripsy; for example, lithotripsy: _____. (*p. 454*)
    1. A closing
    2. A widening
    3. A crushing
    4. A reduction

23. -uria; for example, albuminuria: _____. (*p. 454*)
    1. Stone
    2. Urine
    3. Reduction
    4. Enlargement

5.3 THE AGING PROCESS AS IT RELATES TO DISEASES COMMON TO THE NURSING HOME POPULATION

1. The bones, muscles, cartilage, tendons, and joints used in movement are the: _____. (p. 455)
   1. Nervous system
   2. Respiration
   3. Reproductive
   4. Musculoskeletal system

2. The system that circulates blood is also called the _____. (p. 456)
   1. Gastric system
   2. Defense system
   3. Cardiovascular system
   4. The nervous system

3. When the health of cells has deteriorated, it usually is due to a decrease in effectiveness of the _____, interfering with the supply of nutrients to them. (p. 458)
   1. Cardiovascular system
   2. Nervous system
   3. Musculoskeletal system
   4. Regenerative capacities

4. A stroke occurs when the lack of oxygen to an area of the brain causes _____. (p. 461)
   1. Insomnia
   2. Increased olfactory acuity
   3. Ductless gland system
   4. Permanent damage

5. An elderly person whose blood pressure is consistently greater than 160/95 is considered to have _____. (p. 464)
   1. Hypertension
   2. A severe stroke
   3. A strong heart
   4. Low blood pressure

6. The left side of the brain controls the functions on the _____ side of the body. (p. 474)
   1. Distal
   2. Front
   3. Left
   4. Right

7. A disease resulting from loss of elasticity in the lung tissues causing carbon dioxide to build up is _____. (p. 470)
   1. Kidney failure
   2. Emphysema
   3. Lung cancer
   4. Pneumonia

8. A progressive disease for which there is no cure, characterized by tremor, rigidity, or muscle stiffness and bradykinesia is _____. (p. 479)
   1. Diverticulitis
   2. Parkinson's disease
   3. Delirium tremens
   4. Crohn's disease

9. Difficulty in swallowing or transferring food from the mouth to the esophagus is called _____. (p. 493)
   1. Esophagitis
   2. Dysphagia
   3. Peptic ulcer
   4. Hiatal hernia

10. The transformation process in which nutrients undergo various chemical reactions is _____. (p. 496)
    1. Dysphagia
    2. Diet
    3. Metabolism
    4. Caloric intake

11. Plasma, which carries red blood cells, and lymph, which carries white blood cells are examples of _____. (p. 497)
    1. Metabolism
    2. Carbohydrates
    3. Body fluids
    4. Liquids

12. Measuring daily fasting blood sugar level and measuring the amount of glucose in the urine are tests used in the treatment of _____. (p. 499)
    1. Diabetes
    2. Acute vitamin deficiencies
    3. Hodgkin's disease
    4. Rheumatic heart disease

13. Infections associated with institutionalization are referred to as _____ infections. (p. 502)
    1. Nosocomial
    2. Internal
    3. Benign
    4. Unnecessary

14. Decubitus ulcers, once formed, can _____. (*p. 505*)
    1. Increase longevity
    2. Become infected and form cavities of dead tissue
    3. Benefit the various organs in the body
    4. Stimulate resident activity

15. The leading types of cancer among males seen in the nursing facility are cancers of the _____. (*p. 511*)
    1. Lung and brain
    2. Prostate gland and rectum
    3. Brain and colon
    4. Lung, colon, and rectum

16. Falls among persons older than 65 years of age account for more than ____% of deaths that result from all falls. (*p. 515*)
    1. 30
    2. 70
    3. 95
    4. 40

17. Chronic renal failure that has progressed to the stage where little or no urine is being produced is called_____. (*p. 520*)
    1. Kidney failure
    2. End-stage renal disease
    3. Renal deficiency
    4. Renal keratosis

18. A study by Stilwell and O'Conner indicated that among persons studied _____. (*p. 526*)
    1. Older people remain interested in sex
    2. Older people find each other attractive
    3. All of these were findings in the Stilwell and O'Conner study
    4. Sexuality contributes to overall well-being

19. The line between disabling mental illnesses and the day-to-day effects of coping with old age _____. (*p. 530*)
    1. Can be readily identified
    2. Is often blurred
    3. Can be measured
    4. Is usually available on the nursing reports

20. In the nursing facility, person-centered administration means focusing on _____. (*p. 533*)
    1. Excellence in pain management
    2. The quality of resident life
    3. Excellence in medication administration
    4. Keeping staff trained

21. The process by which the body breaks down the foods eaten into a form usable by individual cells is _____. (*p. 455*)
    1. Digestion
    2. Dieting
    3. Processing
    4. Metabolism

22. Combined with oxygen, nutrients permit individual cells to perform chemical reactions that _____. (*p. 457*)
    1. Destroy vitamins
    2. Produce energy
    3. Stop chemical reactions
    4. Facilitate chemical reactions

23. Peripheral vascular disease commonly refers to the increased resistance in the blood vessels _____ (*p. 462*)
    1. Primarily in the head
    2. In the chest region
    3. Crohn's disease
    4. In the extremities

24. When the heart muscle itself suffers from a lack of oxygen due to blockages in the arteries that usually supply it, it is known as _____. (*p. 462*)
    1. Coronary artery disease
    2. Decreased blood flow
    3. Decreased blood supply
    4. Progressive organ failure

25. Blood being backed up in the circulatory system causing fluids to leak out of the bloodstream is symptomatic of _____. (*p. 465*)
    1. Risk of heart attack
    2. Anorexia
    3. Congestive heart failure
    4. An aging resident with kidney infection

26. Because tuberculosis can be transmitted through secretions or when a person coughs, it is considered _____. (*p. 472*)
    1. An old person's disease
    2. The onset of methicillin-resistant *Staphylococcus aureus* (MRSA)
    3. An infectious disease
    4. A lung disease

27. The primary problem resulting in glaucoma is _____. (*p. 475*)
    1. Pressure due to failure of fluids to drain normally
    2. Reduction in the level of aqueous humor
    3. Changes in the retina
    4. Shrinkage of the lens of the eye

28. The digestive system is referred to as the alimentary tract or the _____. (*p. 490*)
    1. The digestive tract
    2. Upper and lower intestine
    3. Bowels
    4. Gastrointestinal tract

29. Sharp burning abdominal pain 1 to 4 hours after eating, nausea, weight loss, and blood in stools can be symptoms of _____. (*p. 494*)
    1. Increased risk of stroke
    2. Fats
    3. Excessive protein
    4. An ulcer

30. Carbohydrates can be broken down readily into fuel for the body. Two common sources are _____. (*p. 496*)
    1. Starches and sugars
    2. Minerals and vitamins
    3. Sodium and its substitutes
    4. Calcium and iron

31. During the years 1993 to 2006, the percent of residents in U.S. nursing facilities who had psychological diagnoses _____. (*p. 482*)
    1. Increased
    2. Remained steady
    3. Declined
    4. Rose, then fell back

32. Gastrostomy tubes for residents needing long-term tube feeding may be preferred over nasogastric tubes because there is no chance that fluids may be _____. (*p. 498*)
    1. Leaked
    2. Overcontrolled
    3. Lost
    4. Aspirated

33. Diabetes occurs when the body is unable to metabolize _____ because of a problem with a hormone called insulin. (*p. 499*)
    1. Vitamins
    2. Minerals
    3. Glucose
    4. Potassium

34. Anemia occurs when there is a difficulty with the _____ blood cells resulting in the body not getting enough oxygen. (*p. 499*)
    1. White
    2. Red
    3. White and red
    4. Disease fighting

35. The skin, the acid composition of gastric juices, and the urine are _____ that help to protect the body. (*p. 501*)
    1. Barrier-type defenses
    2. Ineffective-type defenses
    3. Immune defenses
    4. Internal organs

36. Whenever foreign material or _____ enter the body, the components of the immune system recognize this and mobilize for an attack response. (*p. 501*)
    1. Antighesis
    2. Antigens
    3. Antidotes
    4. Antibacterials

37. Redness surrounding the areas of skin that may become infected is called the _____ response. (*p. 503*)
    1. Action
    2. Antiallergic
    3. Offense
    4. Inflammation

38. The tough, dry, wrinkled skin sometimes observed among elderly persons may work to _____ the barrier effect of the skin. (*p. 503*)
    1. Improve
    2. Diminish
    3. Rejuvenate
    4. Heighten

39. The formation of a skin ulcer can occur when _____. (*p. 505*)
    1. The body's chemical defense mechanism suddenly degrades
    2. The weight of the body exerts unusual pressure on internal soft tissue
    3. Patients reach advanced age
    4. Patients' diets are altered

40. Residents most at risk of developing pressure sores are those _____. (*p. 505*)
    1. With poor personal hygiene
    2. With excessive fat tissue
    3. Who have poor dentition
    4. Who are immobile

41. The percentage of U.S. nursing home residents who were chairbound in 2013 was just more than ____ (*p. 507*)
    1. 95%
    2. 9%
    3. 25%
    4. 50%

42. Hypothermia is often difficult to diagnose because symptoms may be similar to _____. (*p. 509*)
    1. Mild anorexia
    2. A minor stroke
    3. A massive heart attack
    4. Advanced cancer symptoms

43. The proportion of residents in U.S. nursing facilities during 1993 to 2013 who received special skin care _____. (*p. 508*)
    1. More than doubled
    2. Remained the same
    3. Decreased
    4. Increased fourfold

44. Joints are the points in the body at which _____. (*p. 512*)
    1. Bones are always fused
    2. The ends of two bones meet
    3. Breaks have earlier occurred
    4. Ulcers form

45. There is some consensus among researchers that during the aging process the total amount of bone in the body _____. (*p. 512*)
    1. Decreases
    2. Increases
    3. Becomes elevated
    4. Remains stable

46. The proportion of residents in U.S. nursing homes during 1993 to 2013 who were incontinent remained about _____. (*p. 521*)
    1. More than 90%
    2. Too few to meaningfully measure
    3. About 10%
    4. 50%

47. Orthostatic hypotension is _____. (*p. 443*)
    1. Decreased blood pressure on standing
    2. Excessive irritability
    3. Decreased irritability
    4. Degenerative bone disease leading to weakening of the bones

48. In addition to removing waste materials from the bloodstream, the kidneys also help to regulate the _____. (*p. 518*)
    1. Amount of body fluids
    2. Ductless gland system
    3. Pituitary gland
    4. Thalamus gland

49. Itchy and dry skin, mental confusion, weakness, muscle cramps, nausea, vomiting, and diarrhea can all be the symptoms of _____. (*p. 520*)
    1. Oncoming chronic renal failure
    2. Hyperactive kidneys
    3. Excessive rate of urine production
    4. Constant urine production

50. Patients unable to urinate can be _____ periodically following fluid intake. (*p. 522*)
    1. Advised
    2. Ambulated
    3. Catheterized
    4. Rejoined

51. During midlife, women experience cessation of egg production, and hence of menstruation, called _____. (*p. 525*)
    1. Menopause
    2. Hysterectomy
    3. Genital prolapse
    4. Prostatitis

52. An elderly male nursing facility resident with painful urination and blood in the urine should be checked for _____. (*p. 526*)
    1. Rectal cancer
    2. Dermal cancer
    3. Prostatitis
    4. Dysphagia

53. The incidence of heart attack or stroke during sexual intercourse _____. (*p. 527*)
    1. Is a major concern for nursing home physicians
    2. Has been identified as a valid health issue
    3. Is very low
    4. Has been declining during the past decade

54. Fantasizing, avoidance of eye contact, fidgeting, insomnia, isolation from others, and hostile or dependent behaviors are thought to be manifestations of _____. (*p. 528*)
    1. Personal abilities
    2. Repressive staff
    3. Anxiety
    4. Exploratory behavior

55. Psychotropic drugs exert an effect primarily on the _____. (*p. 529*)
    1. Brain
    2. Digits
    3. Internal organs
    4. Extremities

56. Nearly _____ of all residents in U.S. nursing homes in 2006 were receiving psychoactive drugs. (*p. 530*)
1. 10%
2. One quarter
3. Three fourths
4. Two thirds

57. There are losses incoming residents inevitably experience, and _____. (*p. 434*)
1. These can never be understood
2. They are most difficult to identify
3. There are also gains
4. They are quickly forgotten

58. Anger and anxiety typically associated with being admitted to a nursing facility can lead to _____ (*p. 530*)
1. An easy adjustment
2. Admission-associated depression
3. Hyperactivity
4. Relief

59. The number of facilities receiving citations for improper restraint use in 2006 was about_____ than in 1993. (*p. 532*)
1. 5% less
2. One third less
3. Out of proportion
4. Dramatically more

60. Experience suggests that it is important to identify depression on top of _____. (*p. 532*)
1. Dementia
2. Advanced psychosis
3. Early Alzheimer's
4. Advanced Alzheimer's

61. Among persons aged 65 years, _____ is/are the ninth leading cause of death and the leading cause of fatal and nonfatal injuries. (*p. 515*)
1. Decubitus ulcers
2. Bad judgment
3. Poor eyesight
4. Falls

62. The most effective fall intervention strategy is a _____ fall-risk reduction program for each resident based on paying careful attention to the comprehensive assessment of each resident. (*p. 515*)
1. Well-developed facility program
2. Facility staff attention to
3. Personalized
4. Standardized and enforced

63. ■ To begin as early as possible (first 24–48 hours)
    ■ To assess the patient systematically (first 2–7 days)
    ■ To prepare the therapy plan carefully
    ■ To build up in stages
    ■ To include the type of rehabilitation approach specific to deficits

    These are the basic principles of _____ (*pp. 517–518*)
    1. Nursing care
    2. Hospice care
    3. Rehabilitation
    4. Occupational therapy

64. Vital signs, galvanic skin responses, heart rate variations and recovery, patterns of communication, movement and activity, posture, quality and duration of sleep and brain waves _____. (*p. 529*)
    1. Define depression
    2. Cause resident blues
    3. Can track depression
    4. Are precursors to depression

Facility Policies

Putting the Systems Together

6.1 SETTING POLICIES FOR THE FACILITY

6.1.1 ADMINISTRATION POLICIES

1. If a nursing facility has been certified by Medicare and Medicaid under Final Rules and federal requirements, in effect, it _____. (See Federal Requirements App. P and PP.)* (*p. 542*)**
   1. Can be exempted from state and local licensure requirements
   2. Must still meet all state and local licensure requirements
   3. Is deemed to have met all state and local licensure requirements
   4. May apply for a waiver from state requirements

2. Establishing and implementing policies regarding the management of the facility are assigned to _____. (See Federal Requirements App. P and PP.) (*p. 543*)
   1. The administrator
   2. The owner(s)
   3. The governing body or persons designated as such
   4. The facility staff

3. In order to begin collecting better data about the nursing home industry, federal legislation mandated development and use of _____. (See Federal Requirements App. P and PP.) (*p. 542*)
   1. The Comprehensive Care Approach
   2. A Minimum Data Set
   3. Changes in record keeping
   4. A state-developed data collection system

---

*Answers can be found in *Nursing Home Federal Requirements: Guidelines to Surveyors and Survey Protocols*, Eighth Edition.

**Answers can be found in *Nursing Home Administration*, Seventh Edition, on the page numbers in parentheses following each question.

4. The comprehensive care plan does not include a(an) _____. (See Federal Requirements App. P and PP.) (*p. 580*)
   1. Attending physician
   2. Registered nurse caregiver
   3. Resident
   4. Medical director

5. Nurse's aides who have completed a training and competency evaluation program and passed the required competency test(s) _____. (See Federal Requirements App. P and PP.) (*p. 545*)
   1. May serve at any facility
   2. Must still be judged by surveyors as competent to provide services
   3. May, at their option, be registered with the state nurse's aide registry
   4. May sit for training for nurse's aide assistant, IV

6. Responsibility for ascertaining professional performance standards for licensed, certified, or registered allied health persons used by the facility rests with the _____. (See Federal Requirements App. P and PP.) (*p. 543*)
   1. Respective certifying or registering boards
   2. Resident or the resident's responsible party
   3. State
   4. Facility

7. Organizations that actually pay the Medicare claims submitted by doctors and other medical suppliers are called _____. (See Federal Requirements App. P and PP.) (*p. 348*)
   1. Carriers
   2. Medicare contractors
   3. Third-party payers
   4. Intermediaries

RESOURCE UTILIZATION

8. The facility is not required to use its resources effectively and efficiently to attain the highest practical _____. (*p. 542*)
   1. Resident physical well-being
   2. Resident mental well-being
   3. Profitability
   4. Resident psychosocial well-being

MENTAL ILLNESS

9. A person who is determined by the state mental health authority to need nursing facility service but is receiving active treatment for mental illness _____. (See Federal Requirements App. P and PP.) (*p. 549*)
   1. Can be admitted
   2. Must not be admitted
   3. May be admitted if the medical director authorizes it
   4. Must go to the state mental hospital or equivalent

10. Each facility must designate a physician to serve as medical director _____. (See Federal Requirements App. P and PP.) (*p. 546*)
    1. On a part-time basis
    2. On a full-time basis
    3. On a part- or full-time basis
    4. When needed

COMPLIANCE WITH LAWS

11. The administrator believes that once the obligation to meet federal state and local laws is met, the requirements applicable to the operation of the facility have been satisfied. The administrator is _____. (*p. 542*)
    1. Following all requirements
    2. By definition meeting standards
    3. Exceeding minimum operational standards
    4. Only partially correct

12. The terms for Medicare and Medicaid participating homes used in the Final Rules effect are _____. (See Federal Requirements App. P and PP.) (*p. 343*)
    1. Nursing home and nursing facility
    2. Medicaid facility and Medicare facility
    3. Skilled nursing facility and nursing facility
    4. Approved facility and licensed facility

13. Having a transfer agreement with one or more hospitals is _____. (See Federal Requirements App. P and PP.) (*p. 543*)
    1. Good practice
    2. A risk management measure
    3. A condition of participation requirement
    4. A wise step in preparation for emergency situations

14. Nursing homes are licensed by _____. (See Federal Requirements App. P and PP.) (*p. 542*)
    1. The counties
    2. The states
    3. The federal regional government arms
    4. Centers for Medicare and Medicaid

15. Regulations such as those implementing Medicare and Medicaid; Requirements for Long-Term Care Facilities, are first published in the _____. (See Federal Requirements App. P and PP.) (*p. 542*)
    1. United States Code
    2. National Register
    3. Congressional Record
    4. Federal Register

GOVERNING BODY

16. All facilities are required to _____. (*p. 543*)
    1. Have a governing body
    2. Have an adequately functioning administrator who reports to a corporate board
    3. Have a governing body or designated persons
    4. Have a governing body or designated persons functioning as a governing body

TRANSFER AGREEMENT

17. The facility administrator establishes written transfer agreements with two local hospitals, one of which is approved only for participation under the Medicare program, and the second approved only for participation under Medicaid. The administrator has _____. (*p. 543*)
    1. Failed to meet transfer agreement requirements
    2. Accomplished the minimum required by the Federal Regulations
    3. More than met the minimum required—an agreement with one of these hospitals would meet requirements
    4. Ensured that needed transfers can be accomplished

18. The transfer agreements signed by the administrator ensure that the medical and other information needed for care and treatment of the resident is available and that a bed will be available for the resident on return from the hospital. This is the entire agreement. A visiting surveyor would _____. (*p. 543*)
    1. Find this acceptable
    2. Require changes to the transfer agreement
    3. Believe residents of that facility were being adequately protected
    4. Feel comfortable that a resident's right to return to the facility has been protected

19. The discharge social worker at the hospital determines that the resident cared for under the transfer agreement should return, not to the facility, but be placed in an assisted living facility that is a less expensive setting. Normally, _____ (*p. 543*)
    1. This is inappropriate
    2. This is appropriate
    3. Is outside the prerogative of a hospital
    4. Frowned on by Medicare

CHANGES IN OWNERSHIP

20. If persons with controlling interest in the facility, the company owning the facility, or the administrator or director of nursing change, the facility should_____. (*p. 543*)
    1. Call and inform the state facility licensing agency
    2. Inform the state licensing agency in writing
    3. Inform the Medicare Intermediary
    4. Inform the state Medicaid officials

6.1.2 PERSONNEL POLICIES

Properly Qualified Activities Program Professional

21. The administrator decides the trained therapeutic recreation specialist is too costly for the facility and hires instead a less expensive qualified occupational therapy assistant. This is _____. (*p. 544*)
    1. Within the federal hiring guidelines
    2. Outside the federal hiring guidelines
    3. An unfortunate decision
    4. Likely to not be a cost-effective decision

Social Services

22. The recently graduated social worker job applicant for a 140-bed facility states that she has a bachelor's degree in psychology and 1 year's experience as supervisor of four social workers at a nearby nursing hospital. The administrator should _____. (*p. 545*)
    1. Be satisfied that the applicant meets requirements for the facility
    2. Hire the applicant
    3. Explore the applicant's experience in more depth
    4. Be pleased that the applicant has supervised four social workers

Registered Nurse

23. The administrator of a 50-bed facility asks the director of nursing to serve as both director of nursing and as a charge nurse on the weekend shift. (*p. 545*)
    1. This is appropriate
    2. Minimum staffing has been met
    3. Minimum staffing has not been met
    4. Not permitted

24. If a facility provides the stated minimum number of hours per resident day of care, a state or federal inspector _____. (See Federal Requirements App. P and PP.) (*p. 545*)
    1. May still cite nursing for insufficient staffing
    2. Will pass the facility on staffing
    3. Will require the facility to maintain that ratio
    4. May, at his or her discretion, reduce the staffing required

25. If the administrator of an average daily total occupancy of 80 residents requires the director of nursing to serve as charge nurse, the administrator _____. (See Federal Requirements App. P and PP.) (*p. 545*)
    1. Has met Final Rules requirements
    2. Needs to routinely report the assignment to the state
    3. Has failed to meet Final Rules requirements
    4. Has exceeded Final Rules requirements

Consultant Pharmacist

26. The consultant pharmacist at his monthly visit requires the director of nursing to provide him with a reconciliation report for all controlled drugs signed verified by the director of nursing. The pharmacist _____. (*p. 545*)
    1. Has met his obligations
    2. Has acted in good faith
    3. Should determine himself that drug records are in order
    4. Is meeting the expectations of Medicare and Medicaid record keeping

Training of Nurse's Aides

27. The personnel director recommends a part-time nurse's aide who has worked at the facility for the past 6 months and is nearing the end of her competency evaluation program be hired as a full-time aide. The administrator should feel that the personnel director is _____. (*p. 545*)
    1. Doing a good job
    2. Not understanding the requirements
    3. Smart to have a person under observation for 6 months before permanent hiring
    4. Functioning quite well

Regular In-Service Education

28. At least every 12 months the facility requires all full- and part-time nurse's aides to fill in a report on the continuing education done by each aide in the facility. This report is then filed in the employee's personnel file. The facility is _____. (*p. 545*)
    1. Meeting reporting requirements
    2. Right to keep the signed report in the employee's personnel file
    3. Not keeping adequate records of training
    4. Failing to train based on outcome of these reviews

Use of Outside Resources

29. When the facility does not employ a qualified professional to furnish a service to be provided by the facility, the facility _____. (*p. 546*)
    1. Can provide a list of suitably qualified professionals in the community
    2. Can seek volunteer help for unmet services
    3. Must use the local hospital
    4. Must have that service furnished

Disaster and Emergency Preparedness

30. The facility should train all employees in emergency procedures _____. (*p. 546*)
    1. By the end of the first week on the job
    2. The first day on the job
    3. As soon as training staff are available
    4. Before the employee's first day on the job

31. The facility must train _____ in emergency procedures _____. (*p. 546*)
    1. All caregiver employees/when they begin to work
    2. All employees/when they begin to work
    3. Designated employees/within 3 weeks of employment
    4. New employees/within 1 week

Not Employing Certain Individuals

32. When a facility learns a court of law has taken action against one of its employees indicating unfitness for service, the facility must _____. (*p. 547*)
    1. Fire that employee immediately
    2. Give the employee 2 weeks' notice
    3. Require additional in-service education for that employee
    4. Report the court's action to licensing authorities

33. Ms. Brown alleges for the 12th documented time that she was abused by an employee. The facility _____. (*p. 548*)
1. Is justified in the documenting, but not investigating the matter
2. Is negligent in protecting patients
3. Should counsel with the resident
4. Should consider transferring that resident to a more suitable facility

6.1.3 DIETARY

34. If the facility does not employ a full-time qualified dietitian the facility _____. (*p. 548*)
1. Can appoint instead a full-time director of food services
2. May seek consultation from the outside
3. Designates a director of food services who receives consultation from a qualified dietitian
4. Employees a nutrition expert who advises the director of food service

35. The facility must employ a _____ either full time, part time, or on a consultant basis. (See Federal Requirements App. P and PP.) (*p. 548*)
1. Director of food services
2. Chef
3. Sufficient dietary staff
4. Qualified dietitian

6.1.4 ADMISSIONS POLICIES

36. Orders for routine care or to improve the resident's functional abilities must be available _____. (*p. 548*)
1. At admission
2. Within 24 hours of admission
3. Within 36 hours of admission
4. By the second shift after readmission

6.1.6 REHABILITATION POLICIES

37. If mental health rehabilitative services for mental illness or mental retardation are required in the resident's plan of care, the facility _____. (*p. 550*)
1. May seek to transfer the resident to a mental health services setting
2. Must transfer the resident to a mental health services setting
3. Must provide such services in house
4. Must provide in house or obtain such services

38. The care plan team determines that although they had not anticipated it, the resident needs physical therapy. The facility should _____. (*p. 548*)
1. Assign the therapy to a qualified physical therapist either in house or from outside
2. Get a physician's written order
3. Get authorization from the Medicare provider
4. Begin the physical therapy as soon as possible

6.1.7 RESIDENT'S RIGHTS

Incompetence/Competence

39. A resident who has been determined by the courts to be incompetent decides he no longer wants the court-appointed representative to handle his personal funds and asks the facility to establish a personal funds account for him. The facility should_____. (*p. 557*)
1. Establish a personal funds account for that resident
2. Seek the advice of an attorney
3. Ask the court-appointed representative for permission to establish an account
4. Get the advice of the facility accountant

40. Perhaps the most basic purpose of the new management of personal resident funds rules is to _____. (See Federal Requirements App. P and PP.) (*p. 551*)
1. Reduce resident confusion about finances
2. Improve facility accounting efficiency
3. Improve interest rates to residents by pooling resident funds
4. Avoid commingling resident funds with facility funds

41. Notifying _____ residents when their account reaches _____ less than the _____ resource limit for one person is required. (See Federal Requirements App. P and PP.) (*p. 557*)
1. Medicare/$200/Supplemental Security Income (SSI)
2. Medicaid/$300/Social Security Administration
3. Medicaid/$200/SSI
4. All/$200/personal funds

42. On discovering that the new intake social worker required the individual holding durable power of attorney for a patient's funds to sign a contract guaranteeing payment from that patient's funds, the administrator should _____. (See Federal Requirements App. P and PP.) (*p. 564*)
1. Discourage the social worker from finding similar admissions
2. Revoke the guarantee of payment document
3. Discipline the social worker
4. Praise the intake social worker

43. Rights of residents who are adjudged incompetent by a court are exercised by
_____. (See Federal Requirements App. P and PP.) (*p. 553*)
1. The locally appointed ombudsman
2. The family
3. A person appointed by the court
4. The responsible adult

44. Under the Final Rules, the right to immediate access to any resident by representatives of the state, ombudsman, protection agencies, and advocacy agencies
is _____. (See Federal Requirements App. P and PP.) (*p. 560*)
1. Subject to resident approval
2. Unrestricted
3. Carefully set out as to time and place
4. Subject to facility approval

45. A representative of the state ombudsman office demands to see the clinical
record of a Medicaid resident who had written that he wanted no one to have
access to his clinical record. On receiving the request, you, the administrator,
should _____. (See Federal Requirements App. P and PP.) (*p. 560*)
1. Deny permission to the ombudsman
2. Provide access to the record requested by the ombudsman
3. Tell the ombudsman you will seek legal counsel, then respond
4. Ask the ombudsman to return at a later time

Resident's Exercise of Rights Without Reprisal

46. The resident hangs a religious ornament above her bed. Several nurse's aides
are offended and feel it is inappropriate. The facility administrator should
_____. (*p. 551*)
1. Seek a resident council opinion
2. Advise the aides that this is appropriate
3. Try to enforce the separation of church and state rules
4. Get the facility attorney involved

Resident's Rights to All Records

47. A resident may refuse to release personal and clinical records when _____. (See
Federal Requirements App. P and PP.) (*p. 554*)
1. Transferred to another health care facility
2. Third-party payment contracts seek it
3. Required by law
4. Required by the duly appointed state ombudsman

48. A resident asks the afternoon nurse on duty to access his patient records. The nurse responds that she will have the records made available by late tomorrow morning. The nurse's response is _____. (*p. 554*)
1. A denial of resident rights
2. Appropriate
3. An unpermitted delay
4. Clearly a delaying tactic

49. Congress intends that residents have the right to inspect, on 48 hours' notice, _____. (See Federal Requirements App. P and PP.) (*p. 554*)
1. Their medical record
2. The plan of care
3. Medication records
4. All their records

Resident's Rights to Full Total Health Status Information

50. A resident is concerned about her cognitive status and asks to see all the facility has in her records about her cognitive status including tests administered at admission 4 weeks earlier. The resident is _____. (*p. 554*)
1. Unnecessarily worried
2. Inappropriate
3. Asking for information the facility should withhold
4. Within her rights

51. The new resident speaks only Japanese. Before the resident was admitted, the facility advised him through his interpreter that no one in the facility spoke Japanese and that solely sign language would be used. On examining this admission condition in the resident's records, the surveyor would _____. (*p. 555*) 554
1. Feel the facility had made a reasonable choice
2. Ask to see the signage to assess its adequacy
3. Cite the facility
4. Suggest ways the facility might better communicate with this resident

Resident's Rights to Advance Directives and to Refuse Treatment and/or Research

52. After the first of 10 scheduled physical therapy sessions following her surgery, the resident tells the physical therapist she is not going to keep the final nine appointments. The resident is _____. (*p. 555*)
1. Making a foolish decision
2. Exceeding her rights to control her health care
3. Within her rights
4. Making a questionable decision

53. The resident decides to discontinue all the nine drugs being administered daily. The facility staff feel this may result in a coma likely followed by death. The facility _____. (*p. 555*)
    1. Can modify this decision as needed to keep the resident alive
    2. Must comply and maintain the resident at highest level within that decision
    3. Must contact and follow the physician's orders
    4. Should consider transferring the resident

54. Informing a resident of his rights is required _____. (*p. 556*)
    1. Within 24 hours of admission
    2. Prior to admission
    3. Prior to or at admission
    4. As a courtesy to each entering resident

Work

55. A resident may perform services for the facility if the services are _____. (See Federal Requirements App. P and PP.) (*p. 560*)
    1. Voluntary
    2. Paid at or above prevailing rates
    3. In the plan of care
    4. Light duty in nature

56. When the physician decides to discontinue an existing form of treatment due to adverse consequences, the facility _____. (*p. 557*)
    1. Must note this in the resident's care plan
    2. Must notify the resident and the resident's representative
    3. Inform the pharmacy of this new information
    4. Order new replacement drugs

Protection of Resident's Funds

57. The facility staff suspect family members are abusing a resident's funds and requires that, for the resident's protection, his funds must be deposited with the facility. This is _____. (*p. 557*)
    1. A prudent step for the facility
    2. Not permitted
    3. Subject to review by the owners
    4. A routine protection afforded residents by most facilities

58. A resident routinely maintained $40 in her personal funds account and is upset to learn the facility has her funds in a noninterest-bearing account. Placing this resident's funds in a noninterest-bearing account is_____. (*p. 557*)
    1. Permitted
    2. Required
    3. Optional if the resident agrees
    4. Expected financial behavior

59. A facility that informs each resident who is entitled to Medicaid benefits, in writing, at admission, and when changes of services that are paid for under the State plan occur, has _____. (See Federal Requirements App. P and PP.) (*p. 556*)
    1. Met its obligations
    2. Exceeded its required information
    3. Not fully met its notice of service obligations
    4. Properly interpreted the Final Rules requirement to inform

60. On the death of a Medicaid resident, the facility conveyed the resident's funds within 14 days and promised to forward a final accounting in 3 weeks. This is _____. (*p. 558*)
    1. Within the required notification periods
    2. A failure to meet notification requirements
    3. Faster refunding and accounting than required
    4. Meeting minimum standards

61. As part of a larger chain, the local facility believes that self-insurance plus use of Federal Deposit Insurance Corporation insured accounts is a reasonable protection of resident funds. The surveyor is likely _____. (*p. 558*)
    1. To agree
    2. To want to ensure financial stability by reviewing the balance sheets for the facility
    3. To issue a deficiency
    4. Examine the facility's financial track record

Allowable Charges

62. The facility routinely charges all cosmetic and grooming items and services for private, Medicare, and Medicaid residents. This charging policy _____. (*p. 558*)
    1. Is permitted at facility discretion
    2. Meets Medicare rules, but not Medicaid rules
    3. Meets all rules
    4. Is not permitted for Medicare and Medicaid residents

63. The facility proudly installed flat-screen TVs in all residents' rooms and added a small surcharge to all residents' monthly charges. This freed up significant floor space in each room and improved resident morale. This approach to improving resident life_____. (*p. 559*)
    1. Is appropriate
    2. Violates Medicaid and Medicaid rules
    3. Meets Medicare rules but not those of Medicaid
    4. Meets Medicaid, but not Medicare rules

64. The resident reports the facility to the state for releasing his medical records to the local hospital despite his refusal to release these records when he was transferred to the local hospital. The state is likely to _____. (*p. 559*)
    1. Issue a fine
    2. Inform the resident he has no right to refuse to release his records on transfer
    3. Issue a citation
    4. Assure the resident it will not happen again

65. The resident has complained numerous times about the disruptive behavior of a nearby resident. The facility assures the resident that nothing can be done. This is_____. (*p. 559*)
    1. Probably an accurate statement by the facility
    2. An inadequate facility response
    3. A routine occurrence
    4. Not addressed by federal rules

66. A resident demands to see both the most recent survey results and the plan of correction. The facility shows the survey results, but tells the resident that the plan of correction is confidential and not available. The facility is _____. (*p. 559*)
    1. Within its rights
    2. Violating resident rights
    3. Acting prudently
    4. Protecting sensitive information

Work

67. The resident requested work delivering newspapers throughout the facility. This is an approved part of the resident's care plan. The resident receives $5.00 an hour for this work. The facility is _____. (*p. 560*)
    1. Meeting work requirements
    2. Not meeting work requirements
    3. Improperly documenting the resident's work
    4. Appropriately humoring the resident

Mail Rights in Sending and Receiving

68. The resident demands computer and Internet access, but the facility fails to provide this. The facility _____. (*p. 560*)
    1. Is within its rights
    2. Is failing to meet requirements
    3. Behind the times
    4. Worried about resident privacy

Access and Visitation Rights

69. A representative of the secretary knocks on the locked front door at 5:30 a.m. and wants immediate admission. The charge nurse tells the representative to wait until the facility opens at 6:00 a.m. This is_____. (*p. 560*)
    1. Within the facility's discretion
    2. Good judgment
    3. A safety and risk management behavior
    4. A violation

Furniture

70. The administrator refuses to permit a large piece of furniture to be placed in the resident's room arguing that it overly obstructs movement. The administrator is _____. (*p. 570*)
    1. Within her rights
    2. Ignoring resident rights
    3. Making her own rules without regard to the resident
    4. Making a mistake

Married Couples Sharing a Room

71. Consenting married residents have a right to share a room_____. (*p. 561*)
    1. Regardless of their health conditions
    2. If facility policy permits
    3. When a room is conveniently available
    4. When approved by the resident council

Self-Administration of Drugs (Requirements)

72. An individual resident can self-administer drugs if _____. (*p. 561*)
    1. The pharmacy approves
    2. The attending physician approves
    3. The interdisciplinary team has determined this is safe
    4. The resident accepts responsibility for storing the drugs safely

Resident Transfers

73. The facility may transfer a resident_____. (*p. 562*)
    1. When beds are scarce
    2. When the resident is a month late in payment of charges
    3. If the facility will close within 1 year
    4. If the resident is persistently disruptive to other patients' comfort

74. The facility seeking to transfer a resident must _____. (*p. 562*)
1. Record the reasons in the resident's clinical record
2. Give 90 days' notice
3. Have a good reason
4. Need the bed for an other resident who is returning from the hospital

75. When a facility notifies a resident of a transfer on February 1, to be accomplished March 1, the facility has _____. (See Federal Requirements App. P and PP.) (*p. 563*)
1. Met Final Rules requirements
2. Failed to meet Final Rules requirements
3. Taken appropriate action when unable to meet needs
4. Acted in good faith

76. When the nurse gives complete verbal notice of the duration of the bed-hold policy under the state plan to a resident and his family before transfer to a hospital, the facility can be said to have _____. (See Federal Requirements App. P and PP.) (*p. 563*)
1. Met Final Rules requirements
2. Failed to meet Final Rules requirements
3. Exceeded Final Rules requirements
4. Conformed acceptably to Final Rules requirements

Family Meetings

77. Regarding group or family meetings, after providing space and privacy to resident families and any invited persons, the facility obligations are _____. (See Federal Requirements App. P and PP.) (*p. 567*)
1. Met
2. Partially met
3. Exceeded
4. Optional as to further assistance

Private Pay

78. The facility is by policy a 100% private pay residents' facility. The facility informs prospective residents of this both in writing and orally in a language they can understand. This_____. (*p. 556*)
1. Meets the facility's obligations
2. Is permitted under special circumstances in some Medicare-certified facilities
3. Is not permitted
4. Is a safe business practice

Payments

79. The facility requires only private paying patients to designate a third party who will pay the bills. Medicare and Medicaid patients are billed only from their own funds. This_____. (*p. 556*)
    1. Is a correct interpretation the rules
    2. Is a necessary business practice
    3. Ensures a good collection rate
    4. Violates Medicare and Medicaid standards

Freedom From Restraints

80. The new administrator announces that after 2 weeks, no restraints will be allowed, even those required to meet the residents' medical symptoms. This is _____. (*p. 584*)
    1. Permitted
    2. Not permitted
    3. A violation of federal rules
    4. A misinterpretation of the rules' intent

Abuse

81. To lessen the risk and incidence of residents' abusive treatment of other residents, the facility permits a resident to remain in his room throughout the day. This is _____. (*p. 552*)
    1. Good risk management
    2. Within the intent of the federal rules
    3. Abusive treatment
    4. A good way to reduce incidents of residents abusing other residents

Restraints

82. The administrator who learns that the director of nursing obtained physician's orders for physical restraints on three "too time-consuming 'wanderer'" residents should _____. (See Federal Requirements App. P and PP.) (*p. 552*)   531-532
    1. Compliment the director of nursing on solving a staffing problem
    2. Seek the same for additional residents
    3. Ask the physicians to remove the restraint orders
    4. Continue about her normal daily duties

83. An alleged violation of neglect of a resident has been lodged. The administrator has reported this to the state, conducted an investigation the next day, and concluded no violation occurred. The administrator should _____. (See Federal Requirements App. P and PP.) (*p. 552*)
    1. Report results to state officials within 5 days of the alleged violation
    2. Document the investigation results and file it for state review at annual inspection time
    3. Reprimand the employee involved
    4. Consider the matter successfully settled

6.1.8 QUALITY ASSESSMENT AND ASSURANCE: MEETING THE HOLISTIC NEEDS OF THE CARE RECIPIENTS

84. The facility sets up mechanisms to listen to the views and to record grievances and recommendations of residents and families concerning a proposed policy. The facility has _____. (*p. 567*)
    1. Met expectations under the federal regulation
    2. Exceeded what it is required to do
    3. Failed to meet regulations
    4. Set up a good feedback mechanism

85. A uniform data set describing the resident's capability to perform daily life functions and functional impairments is known as _____. (See Federal Requirements App. P and PP.) (*p. 566*)
    1. The uniform (minimum) (comprehensive) data set
    2. Comprehensive care plan
    3. Resident needs assessment
    4. Resident data assessment card

86. Resident assessments must be conducted within _____ days after admission, after a significant mental or physical change, and at least every _____ months. (See Federal Requirements App. P and PP.) (*p. 579*)
    1. 6/8
    2. 4/6
    3. 14/12
    4. 4/24

87. The resident assessment must be conducted or at least coordinated by and signed by _____. (See Federal Requirements App. P and PP.) (*p. 579*)
    1. The resident's physician
    2. The medical director or resident's physician
    3. A registered nurse
    4. The director of nursing

88. A resident enters a facility continent. Due to new clinical conditions catheterization becomes necessary. The facility's entire response is to provide services "to prevent urinary tract infections" and treat them if occurring. The facility has _____. (See Federal Requirements App. P and PP.) (*p. 582*)
    1. Met Final Rules standards
    2. Failed to meet Final Rules standards
    3. Exceeded what is required under Final Rules
    4. Performed good quality care

89. A resident's clinical condition demonstrates that a nasogastric tube is unavoidable. The facility documents this and begins a permanent program designed to prevent aspiration pneumonia, diarrhea, vomiting, dehydration, metabolic abnormalities, and nasal–pharyngeal ulcers. A Medicare inspector would consider the facility to have _____. (See Federal Requirements App. P and PP.) (*p. 582*) 583
    1. Met Final Rules requirements
    2. Exceeded Final Rules requirements
    3. Given excellent care
    4. Failed to implement the intent and spirit of Final Rules

Roommate and Room Changes

90. To accommodate a resident returning from the hospital, the facility informs Mrs. Brown that in half an hour the staff will be moving in a new roommate. The facility _____. (*p. 557*)
    1. Is making the right decision
    2. Has the right to make such needed changes
    3. Is meeting its obligations to residents
    4. Is failing to meet its obligations to residents

Quality Assessment and Assurance

91. The facility appoints the director of nursing, the medical director's physician assistant, and four additional staff members to serve on the Quality Assessment and Assurance Committee. This _____. (*p. 567*)
    1. Meets requirements
    2. Exceeds requirements
    3. Is optional for the facility under the new guidelines
    4. Fails to satisfy the federal guidelines

92. The Quality Assessment and Assurance Committee chair informs the administrator that the committee meets every 4 months and has developed and implemented appropriate plans of action. The administrator should _____. (*p. 568*)
    1. Be pleased
    2. Review the written reports of this committee
    3. Be concerned
    4. Thank the chair

93. During a Medicare survey, the director of nursing refuses to disclose the records of the Quality Assessment and Assurance Committee to enable the surveyor to review the actions taken. The director of nursing is _____. (*p. 568*)
    1. Within her rights
    2. Acting foolishly
    3. Likely to cause an unnecessary deficiency to be given
    4. Using poor judgment

6.1.9 DIETARY

94. The facility identifies low potassium as a nutritional problem, and provides a therapeutic diet to correct the potassium deficiency. The resident refuses the therapeutic diet and insists that he wishes to eat a regular diet just like the other residents. The facility should _____. (*p. 568*)
    1. Serve the therapeutic diet
    2. Serve an enriched diet
    3. Serve a regular diet
    4. Have the resident's attending physician explain why the therapeutic diet is necessary

95. In January, Mrs. Green weighed 112 pounds. In June, she weighed 98 pounds. This is _____. (*p. 568*)
    1. Within normal weight expectations
    2. A significant weight loss
    3. A predictable weight loss
    4. A severe weight loss

Substitutes

96. Mrs. Gray refused to eat the meat served for lunch. The facility offered Mrs. Brown a second salad. This is _____. (*p. 569*)
    1. Within the rules
    2. Appropriate
    3. Inappropriate
    4. Using good judgment because Mrs. Gray is known to especially like salads

97. The registered dietitian prescribes a therapeutic diet for Mrs. Blue because the dietitian noticed some weight loss in the past 2 months. As lunch was about to be served anyway the kitchen staff was able to implement the new diet within 10 minutes of the nutritionist's recommendation. The administrator should _____. (*p. 569*)
    1. Feel his staff is really agile
    2. Meet with the dietitian
    3. Use this as an example of quick work at the next staff meeting
    4. Turn his attention to more pressing matters

98. During the periodic mid-afternoon visit, the consultant dietitian writes out therapeutic diets for the four new residents and hands them as soon as she writes them to the director of food services for those residents that evening. On being informed of this, that afternoon the administrator should _____. (See Federal Requirements App. P and PP.) (*p. 569*)
1. Thank the dietitian for such fast turnaround
2. Check the diets prescribed by the dietitian against the recommended nutritional needs in the Final Rules requirements
3. Tell the director of food services to serve regular diets to those four new residents that night
4. Permit the director of food service 2 days to implement the therapeutic diets

99. Snacks at bedtime _____. (See Federal Requirements App. P and PP.) (*p. 569*)
1. May be offered to competent residents
2. Must be offered to all residents
3. Must be nutritional if offered
4. Must meet Final Rules specified nutritional values

6.1.10 ENVIRONMENTAL MANAGEMENT

Preventive Maintenance

100. The air conditioning roof unit fan shaft has run dry and required repeated quick oiling for several months. The facility is ____. (*p. 571*)
1. Due for a new roof unit
2. Being economical
3. Practicing just-in-time repair
4. Failing to do preventive maintenance

101. A facility initially certified under Final Rules, which at the request of the resident council, maintains a winter temperature of 83° despite protests from staff that this is too hot for the staff is _____. (See Federal Requirements App. P and PP.) (*p. 571*)
1. Complying with Final Rules directives
2. Not in noncompliance with Final Rules
3. Correctly responding to resident directives
4. Voluntarily exceeding the need to acceptably meet resident needs

102. The resident has mentioned to the administrator several times that he is tired of waiting for a room with a window to the outside. The facility is _____. (*p. 573*)
1. Failing to meet physical building requirements
2. Justified if no other rooms are available
3. Not doing enough to meet expectations of residents
4. Needing better policies on meeting resident room preferences

103. Each resident room must have _____. (See Federal Requirements App. P and PP.) (*p. 573*)
    1. A full bath
    2. 125-square feet per resident
    3. Its own fire extinguishment system
    4. At least one window to the outside

104. The call systems representative's recommendations for installing a call system to the bathing facilities in addition to the present resident rooms and toilets call systems were turned down by the administrator as too expensive. This _____. (*p. 573*)
    1. Is the administrator's prerogative
    2. Is reasonable in light of reimbursement levels
    3. Meets enough requirements without the additional call system
    4. Is not meeting standards

6.1.11 INFECTION CONTROL

105. The facility has an infection control program that has effectively investigated and controlled every infectious outbreak. When the state visits and evaluates this program, the state will likely _____. (*p. 574*)
    1. Be pleased
    2. See this as an example to be recommended
    3. Issue a deficiency
    4. Ask about how this has been so successfully accomplished

106. Such details as size of committee, scope of work, and reporting requirements for the infection control function are _____. (See Federal Requirements App. P and PP.) (*p. 574*)
    1. Carefully described in Final Rules
    2. Left to the facility
    3. Left to the individual states to specify
    4. Recommended but not required under Final Rules

107. Maintaining a record of incidents and corrective actions related to infections is assigned under Final Rules to _____. (See Federal Requirements App. P and PP.) (*p. 574*)
    1. The nursing department
    2. The medical director
    3. The infection control program
    4. A mandated quality control coordinator

108. The general approach of the Federal Requirements is to state federal requirements, for example, infection control and budgets, _____. (See Federal Requirements App. P and PP.) (*p. 574*)
1. In general (less specific or detailed) terms
2. In great detail
3. To achieve closer control
4. To ensure identical policies facility to facility

6.1.12 PHYSICIAN SERVICES

109. The nurse was miffed that she could not get a medical decision until the attending physician returns from a medical convention and mentions this to the administrator. The administrator should _____. (*p. 575*)
1. Meet immediately with the director of nursing
2. Assure the resident a decision is being made as soon as practicable
3. Reprimand the nurse
4. Suggest the nurse improve her self-control

110. A physician visit that occurred 14 days after the date the visit was required is _____. (See Federal Requirements App. P and PP.) (*p. 575*)
1. Not considered timely
2. Considered timely
3. Permitted occasionally
4. Routinely permitted

111. If a facility's policy prohibits use of physician assistants, but three physicians routinely use physician assistants for most visits, the Medicare inspector will _____. (See Federal Requirements App. P and PP.) (*p. 576*)
1. Approve the procedure as a Medicare-authorized care procedure
2. Cite the facility
3. Ascertain the acceptability to the residents concerned about the use of physician assistants
4. Encourage such cost savings to Medicare

112. Ultimate responsibility for obtaining and reporting laboratory, radiology, and other diagnostic services is assigned to the _____. (See Federal Requirements App. P and PP.) (*p. 577*)
1. Medical director
2. Nursing facility
3. Attending physician issuing the orders
4. Attending physician's office staff

113. The charge nurse notices that lab work recommended for a particular medication has not been ordered and places the order. The administrator should _____. (See Federal Requirements App. P and PP.) (*p. 577*)
1. Sign off on the order
2. Praise the nurse
3. Document the order
4. Be upset

114. A facility need not first consult with the resident or the resident's physician when there is _____. (See Federal Requirements App. P and PP.) (*p. 576*)
1. An accident involving injury
2. A decision to transfer
3. A change in roommate
4. A medical emergency

115. The medical director declined to take responsibility for monitoring and ensuring implementation of resident care policies feeling this was too time-consuming. The administrator would be well advised to _____. (*p. 576*)
1. Agree with the medical director
2. Enter a complaint to the state about the medical director
3. Find a new medical director
4. Assign that task to the director of nursing

116. On learning that, to save expenses, the director of nursing has determined that drug records are in order and that all controlled drugs are accounted for, the administrator should _____. (See Federal Requirements App. P and PP.) (*p. 577*)
1. Be pleased and compliment the director of nursing
2. Thank the director of nursing for the information and continue about his or her business
3. Call the consulting pharmacist
4. Plan an in-service for other nurses

117. Permitting a resident, whose physician permits drugs judged unnecessary but demanded by the resident, to continue to take unnecessary drugs _____. (See Federal Requirements App. P and PP.) (*p. 585*)
1. Is encouraged
2. Is generally acceptable
3. Is not permitted
4. Is permitted if the resident self-administers drugs

118. New facilities certified under Final Rules must meet the applicable provisions of the _____. (See Federal Requirements App. P and PP.) (*p. 383*)
1. National Fire Protection Association
2. Occupational Safety and Health Act as amended
3. *Life Safety Code*® of 2000
4. *Life Safety Code*® of 1990

Plan D

119. Plan D, implemented in 2006, was intended to _____. (See Federal Requirements App. P and PP.) (*p. 348*)
    1. Provide stricter oversight of care
    2. Provide relief from medication expenses
    3. Cover outlier costs
    4. Decrease federal involvement

Nurse's Aide Training

120. An individual who can prove that he or she recently successfully completed a training and competency evaluation program, but who is not actually registered in the required registry _____ as a nurse's aide. (See Federal Requirements App. P and PP.) (*p. 545*)
    1. Can be hired
    2. Must not be hired
    3. Is temporarily eligible for hiring
    4. Is likely overqualified

121. Responsibility for determining whether the nurse's aide training and competency evaluation requirements are met in a facility falls to the _____. (See Federal Requirements App. P and PP.) (*p. 545*)
    1. Medicare inspectors
    2. Medicaid inspectors
    3. State Nursing Board
    4. State survey agency

122. The owner of a facility providing nearly the best nurse's aide training and competency evaluation program in the state declines to permit an unannounced visit by the state. The state will _____. (See Federal Requirements App. P and PP.) (*p. 545*)
    1. Return at a more acceptable time
    2. Withdraw approval of the training program
    3. Make an announced visit within 5 working days
    4. Make an announced visit within 10 working days

123. The required curriculum for a nurse's aide training program does not have to include _____. (See Federal Requirements App. P and PP.) (*p. 545*)
    1. Basic nursing skills
    2. Personal care skills
    3. Care of cognitively impaired residents
    4. Diet management

124. Candidates for nurse's aide competency evaluation are normally examined by
_____. (See Federal Requirements App. P and PP.) (*p. 545*)
1. A Medicare participating skilled nursing facility
2. A Medicaid nursing facility
3. The individual's own facility
4. A state-approved entity

125. Under federal guidelines, a candidate for nurse's aide registration has _____
chances to take the evaluation. (See Federal Requirements App. P and PP.)
(*p. 545*)
1. Two
2. No more than three
3. Four
4. At least three

126. A finding by the state survey agency of abuse or neglect by a nurse's aide
remains recorded in the nurse's aide registry _____. (See Federal Requirements
App. P and PP.) (*p. 547*)
1. For 2 years
2. For 4 years
3. Forever
4. During the recommended probation period

127. Ensuring that nurse's aides are able to demonstrate competency in skills and
techniques necessary to care for residents' needs is the responsibility of _____.
(See Federal Requirements App. P and PP.) (*p. 545*)
1. The state
2. Medicaid program officials
3. Medicare officials
4. The facility

6.1.13 DENTAL CARE

128. Under Final Rules, routine and emergency dental services are _____. (See
Federal Requirements App. P and PP.) (*p. 578*)
1. Optional
2. Mandated
3. On request of the resident
4. On order of the resident's physician

6.1.14 NURSING REQUIREMENTS

129. The director of nursing mentions to the administrator that although Ms. Brown had no significant change in her physical or mental condition on readmission, a full comprehensive assessment was completed within 5 days of her return. The administrator might feel _____. (*p. 579*)
    1. Facility resources might not be being utilized efficiently
    2. Satisfied that effectiveness had been achieved
    3. Pleased that the assessment was within the 14-day window
    4. Alarmed

130. To stretch resources, the care planning team decides to conduct comprehensive assessments on the healthiest patients every 15 months. The administrator should feel_____. (*p. 579*)
    1. That the staff is making a reasonable choice
    2. The staff is being proactive
    3. A deficiency is in the future
    4. The care team has saved the facility some expenditures

Standards of Quality

131. Standards of quality for care given in the nursing facility _____. (*p. 581*)
    1. May be found in several venues
    2. Come only from the Centers for Medicare and Medicaid (CMS)
    3. Are those set out in the Federal Requirements
    4. Can be developed by the facility or its parent body

6.1.15 QUALITY OF CARE USING THE RESIDENT ASSESSMENT INSTRUMENT TO ENSURE CARE RECIPIENT SATISFACTION

132. The nurse on duty has informed Ms. Brown that Ms. Brown must make arrangements for transportation to her audiologist. This is_____. (*p. 582*)
    1. Correct
    2. Not permitted facility policy
    3. Prudent shepherding of facility staff time
    4. A realistic response

133. Psychosocial adjustment difficulties _____. (*p. 582*)
    1. Are inevitable
    2. Are not common in today's environment
    3. Are the responsibility of the resident
    4. Must be treated by the facility

134. For several months in succession, it is noted in the resident's records that the resident is becoming more withdrawn. The facility _____. (*p. 582*)
    1. Has met its recordkeeping requirements
    2. Should show more staff interest in this resident
    3. Must develop a plan of care to address this
    4. Should provide more opportunities for interaction among the residents

135. For nasogastrically fed patients, the facility program is to provide treatment and services to prevent aspiration, pneumonia, diarrhea, vomiting dehydration, and metabolic abnormalities. This is _____. (*p. 583*)
    1. Satisfactory
    2. More than required
    3. Meets minimum standards
    4. Insufficient

136. Ms. Green has been shouting incoherently at nearby residents. Her physician prescribes an antipsychotic drug to calm her down. This _____. (*p. 585*)
    1. Is reasonable
    2. Is necessary for the comfort of the other residents
    3. Is unacceptable
    4. Follows usual medical practice decisions

6.1.16 PHARMACY

137. The facility must provide a separate, locked, permanently affixed compartment for storage of controlled drugs listed in Schedule _____ of the Drug Act. (*p. 588*)
    1. I
    2. II
    3. III
    4. V

138. Controlled drugs listed in Schedule I of the Comprehensive Drug Abuse Act of 1970 are _____. (See Federal Requirements App. P and PP.) (*p. 588*)
    1. To be kept locked
    2. To be kept locked and under proper temperature controls
    3. Not permitted in the facility
    4. Used only on the order of a licensed physician

6.1.17 MEDICAL RECORDS

139. The administrator's policy is to discard all clinical records after 10 years. This policy is _____. (*p. 588*)
    1. In accordance with requirements
    2. Practical and meets all possible state and federal requirements
    3. Flawed
    4. Causing unduly long retention of records

6.2 DEVELOPING A PERSON-CENTERED CARE PLAN

Resident Assessment Instrument

MDS?

140. The Resident Assessment Instrument is a set of screening, clinical, and functional status elements, which forms the basis for _____. (*p. 589*)
    1. A comprehensive assessment of each resident   *590*
    2. A thorough plan of care
    3. Improving reimbursement
    4. Capacity for a look-back in care needs

141. Specific resident responses for one or a combination of Minimum Data Set (MDS) elements are _____. (*p. 590*)
    1. The minimum elements
    2. The Resident Assessment Instrument (RAI)
    3. The Care Area Triggers
    4. The care plan

142. The Minimum Data Set (MDS) care planning process can be visualized as: assessment, decision making, and _____. (*p. 590*)
    1. Follow-up
    2. Visualization of resident needs
    3. Documentation of resident preferences
    4. Care plan

6.3 THE QUALITY INDICATORS SURVEY

143. In planning an annual survey, the surveyor begins with reviewing current government data records on the facility, current complaints, Ombudsman information, and _____. (*p. 594*)
    1. The facility care plans
    2. The comprehensive assessments
    3. Current Minimum Data Set (MDS) data
    4. All OSCAR data

144. The surveyors expect information on contact persons for complaints or abuse, a list of ventilator dependent residents, a list of residents on hospice, and a list of dialysis patients within _____ of entering a facility for survey. (*p. 595*)
1. One day
2. One hour
3. Four hours
4. 24 hours

145. The administrator can expect surveyors to generate _____ lists of residents to be interviewed. (*p. 595*)
1. Two
2. Eight
3. Three or more
4. Six

146. As a matter of policy, at the Exit Conference, _____ is(are) invited to attend. (*p. 596*)
1. All resident council members
2. The resident council president
3. Any interested residents
4. Only invited residents

147. If a facility's plan of correction is found unacceptable _____. (*p. 596*)
1. The facility is fined
2. A fast-track process will begin
3. The facility can appeal
4. A new plan of correction must be submitted

148. Normally a plan of correction _____. (*p. 597*)
1. Is accepted by the state
2. Meets requirements
3. Triggers a revisit
4. Is appealed

149. Hoping to delay an enforcement action, the administrator asks for an Informal Dispute Resolution. The administrator _____. (*p. 597*)
1. Does not understand the process
2. Has made a prudent move
3. Is taking advisable defensive action
4. Will likely win at least half the time

6.4 THE REPORT CARD

150. A finding by surveyors that in both wings of the facility, the water to resident rooms and baths is 8 degrees above the upper temperature limit, but that no one had yet been burned would result in a deficiency characterized as _____. (*p. 597*)
1. Broad and high
2. Widespread
3. Widespread, no actual harm with minimum potential for actual harm
4. Widespread, no actual harm with potential for more than minimal harm

6.5 GETTING REIMBURSED FOR CARE GIVEN

THE PROSPECTIVE PAYMENT SYSTEM

151. The Centers for Medicare and Medicaid's (CMS) goal is to reimburse based on how much _____ is required to care for each patient each month. (*p. 599*)
1. Money
2. Staff in place
3. Effort
4. Staff time

152. There are _____ levels and types of care for reimbursing nursing facility care given. (*p. 599*)
1. Increasingly diverse
2. Sixty-six
3. Fifteen
4. Five broad categories of

THE MINIMUM DATA SET (MDS)

153. The Minimum Data Set (MDS) contains items that reflect the _____ of the resident. (*p. 599*)
1. Activity level
2. Ability to pay
3. General circumstances
4. Acuity level

154. The Medicare-required assessments provide information about the clinical condition of beneficiaries. These assessments _____ (*p. 599*)
    1. Can be scheduled in advance
    2. Can be unscheduled
    3. Can be scheduled or unscheduled
    4. Can be known in advance

155. Readmission/return assessment, start of therapy, and end of therapy are _____. (*p. 599*)
    1. Excluded from standardized assessment dates
    2. Standardized assessment dates
    3. The 5-, 14-, 30-, 60-, 90-day assessments
    4. More highly reimbursed

THE RESOURCE UTILIZATION GROUP (RUG) CLASSIFICATION SYSTEM

156. The Resource Utilization Group (RUG)-IV classification system has _____ major categories. (*p. 599*)
    1. Four
    2. Eight
    3. Twelve
    4. A varying number of

157. The scheduled Prospective Payment System (PPS) assessments (performed around days 5, 14, 30, 60, and 90) establish _____ for associated standard payment periods. (*p. 600*)
    1. A little used basis
    2. A free-moving basis
    3. Per-diem payment rates
    4. Monthly rates

ACTIVITIES OF DAILY LIVING (ADLs)

158. The activities of daily living (ADL) score is based on the following ADLs: _____. (*p. 600*)
    1. Bed mobility, activities, toilet use, and ambulating
    2. Transferring, eating, and activities
    3. Walking, bed mobility, and eating
    4. Bed mobility, transfer, toilet use, and eating

REIMBURSEMENT

159. A cancer patient receiving intensive therapies may _____. (*p. 600*)
1. Be a good source of extra revenue
2. Be an ideal admission
3. Cost the facility more than it will be reimbursed
4. Increase facility cash flow positively

160. The current long-term health care delivery system is one in which each player seeks to minimize its own costs at the possible expense of _____. (*p. 600*)
1. The taxpayers
2. Private paying patients
3. The revenue base
4. Other players in the system

161. How much a facility can charge for care given can be characterized as _____. (*p. 601*)
1. A given
2. Easy to chart
3. A simple computer algorithm
4. A moving target

162. Establishing transfer and discharge policies according to the source of payment _____ under Final Rules (See Federal Requirements App. P and PP.) (*p. 562*)
1. Is permitted
2. Is discouraged
3. Is forbidden
4. Must be fully documented

163. The goal of the National Health Care Technology coordinator is to have _____ available to all providers, which can lead to improved quality of care at all levels. (*p. 542*)
1. Interoperable care records
2. Smartphone-based records
3. Universally available records
4. Enlarged records

164. Typically, the responsibility for safety and disaster preparedness falls to the _____. (*p. 546*)
1. Business office
2. Personal services director
3. Administrator
4. Director of nursing

165. Although the drugs in the emergency kit are the pharmacist's responsibility, the _____ using the kit must keep records when each item is used and trigger a reorder as needed to keep the kit fully stocked. (*p. 547*)
1. Nurse's aide
2. Contracted pharmacist's assistant
3. Staff
4. Administrator

166. To the extent possible, ensuring that the facility reflects the culture, ethnicity, race, sexual orientation, gender, religions, and language of the surrounding community is part of _____ (*p. 549*)
1. Diversity awareness
2. Good planning
3. Enlarging the horizons
4. Building better practices

167. _____ is defined as separation of a resident from other residents or from his or her roommate or confinement to his or her room (with or without roommates) against the resident's will, or the will of the resident's legal representative. (*p. 552*)
1. Cordoning off
2. Separating
3. Involuntary seclusion
4. Citizen arrest

168. Ombudspersons _____ direct enforcement authority, but are typically part of the local government structure where their recommendations can carry weight. (*p. 556*)
1. Do not have any
2. Do have
3. May or may not have
4. Usually choose not to exercise

169. In the typical nursing facility, various maintenance and repair services are typically _____, such as grounds maintenance or HVAC (heating and cooling) services and repair. (*p. 572*)
1. Contracted out
2. Done only by facility employees only
3. Shared between nursing and maintenance
4. Always contracted to subcontractors

170. _____ is a portable electronic device that automatically diagnoses the life-threatening cardiac arrhythmias of ventricular fibrillation and ventricular tachycardia in a patient, and is able to treat them through defibrillation. (*p. 580*)
    1. Heart starter machine
    2. Automated external defibrillator (AED)
    3. Emergency medical services (EMS)-only device
    4. Staff friendly device

171. Complaints or accusations of abuse or neglect made by residents or by staff must be _____. (*p. 583*)
    1. Always taken seriously
    2. Reported to staff
    3. Reported to administration
    4. Investigated using a protocol

172. Normally a resident care planning conference is held for each resident at least _____ (*p. 590*)
    1. Quarterly
    2. As needed
    3. Monthly
    4. Semiannually

173. Scope and Severity is a system of rating the seriousness of _____ (*p. 597*)
    1. Poor staff attitudes
    2. Staff attendance
    3. Deficiencies
    4. Restraint reports

Answers and Rationale
for Questions 1 to 31

1. (2) During 1998 and 1999, the price paid per bed in nursing home purchases tended to be too high to sustain over the following years when reimbursements were squeezed by Medicare and Medicaid.

2. (2) It is nearly always desirable to be efficient as well as effective.

3. (2) The administrator fails to anticipate that the occupancy rate of the facility is likely to fall and that, in any case, with the new competition a new approach to admissions will most likely be necessary. The administrator is failing to react appropriately to changes in the environment that will likely impact the facility.

4. (3) From the founding of the large-scale nursing home industry in the 1960s until the year 2000 very few bankruptcies were experienced.

5. (2) Medicare (and Medicaid) forced facilities to give more services for a single reimbursement rate than had been the case previously.

6. (2) Medicare, to cut its own costs, has required facilities to give more services under the Medicare reimbursement given.

7. (4) The director of nursing fails to understand that using expensive RN hours when less expensive licensed practical nurse and certified nurse's assistant hours are the industry standard will be unsustainably expensive for the facility.

8. (4) Case mix in the typical rural facility is hard to manipulate, but in the teaching hospital setting the facility normally must maximize the number of Medicare rehabilitation patients in order to remain competitive and solvent.

9. (4) The director of nursing normally reports directly to the administrator. The assistant administrator wants too much power or does not understand how normal nursing facilities function.

10. (2) Under bankruptcy plans, the court ensures that all current bills are paid. The medical supplies provider does not understand the bankruptcy laws.

11. (3) Leadership by walking around (LBWA), to be effective, must be done daily; weekly is too infrequent.

12. (4) It is normally better to go through the chain of command and let the employees' immediate supervisor request the corrections.

13. (1) A number of market forces have held down any significant building of new facilities in recent years. This may change.

14. (4) The successful nursing home administrator will need to employ several administrative styles to get the facility's work successfully accomplished.

15. (1) This candidate understands the need for flexibility in leadership styles and believes that several styles have been used effectively.

16. (2) Charismatic leadership is given to leaders by followers. A leader cannot just declare himself or herself charismatic.

17. (1) Yes, acute care reimbursement rates are higher than average, but so are the costs!

18. (4) It is impossible to prevent informal communications among nurses. The nurse supervisor does not seem to have enough communication savvy to understand this.

19. (2) The department head understands that employees often engage in selective hearing, that is, hearing good news and screening out anything unpleasant.

20. (4) The administrator must get information from all levels of management in order to know what is actually going on. It is dangerous to rely solely on one person.

21. (4) Nursing shortages come and go, but mostly there is a seemingly chronic shortage of good nurse candidates.

22. (1) It is impossible and undesirable to try to write enough rules to make every facility function successfully.

23. (1) It is normal for the various departments such as nursing, housekeeping, and dietary to seek to "turn over" as much work to other departments as they can.

24. (1) The administrator may have all reports made available to him or her, but requiring that the administrator sees all reports before signing would likely be dysfunctional for getting the facility's work done in a timely manner.

25. (3) Correctly filled-out incident reports are a must for the facility and this situation is not likely to "correct itself" without the administrator's active intervention.

26. (1) Corporate wants that facility to have as nearly a deficiency-free inspection as possible and is willing to pay a little more for that year's performance to achieve this.

27. (1) In recent years, federal and state governments have been seeking to reduce the proportion of funds that go to institutional care.

28. (3) This was a part of the effort a few years ago to get nursing facilities reimbursed for the actual costs incurred in giving care.

29. (2) Expect that efforts to shift cost from Medicare and Medicaid onto facilities will continue.

30. (1) The residents may in fact get better care, but if it is not documented, the survey team has no real way to give credit for the care given. Give excellent care, but also document, document, document.

31. (3) The social worker has to do both if assigned both. The social worker needs to renegotiate the job description with the administrator.

Answer Key

1. NAB DOMAIN: MANAGEMENT, GOVERNANCE, AND LEADERSHIP

LEARNING HOW TO MANAGE THE HEALTH CARE ORGANIZATION

1. 2	32. 3	63. 3	94. 3	125. 3	156. 2	187. 1	218. 4	249. 1
2. 2	33. 3	64. 3	95. 3	126. 2	157. 4	188. 4	219. 2	250. 3
3. 2	34. 4	65. 1	96. 1	127. 3	158. 3	189. 3	220. 2	251. 1
4. 3	35. 3	66. 1	97. 2	128. 2	159. 3	190. 3	221. 2	252. 2
5. 2	36. 4	67. 2	98. 4	129. 4	160. 3	191. 4	222. 2	253. 2
6. 2	37. 1	68. 2	99. 1	130. 4	161. 3	192. 2	223. 3	254. 4
7. 4	38. 3	69. 3	100. 2	131. 3	162. 4	193. 3	224. 3	255. 1
8. 4	39. 3	70. 4	101. 3	132. 4	163. 4	194. 4	225. 1	256. 2
9. 4	40. 3	71. 1	102. 1	133. 3	164. 4	195. 2	226. 3	257. 3
10. 2	41. 2	72. 4	103. 4	134. 3	165. 4	196. 3	227. 2	258. 3
11. 3	42. 3	73. 1	104. 3	135. 1	166. 1	197. 4	228. 3	259. 2
12. 4	43. 2	74. 3	105. 4	136. 3	167. 1	198. 4	229. 3	260. 2
13. 1	44. 3	75. 2	106. 3	137. 2	168. 1	199. 4	230. 3	261. 2
14. 4	45. 2	76. 1	107. 3	138. 3	169. 1	200. 3	231. 3	262. 1
15. 1	46. 4	77. 3	108. 4	139. 2	170. 3	201. 3	232. 1	263. 4
16. 2	47. 3	78. 2	109. 3	140. 3	171. 4	202. 4	233. 3	264. 3
17. 1	48. 1	79. 3	110. 3	141. 4	172. 3	203. 4	234. 3	265. 4
18. 4	49. 2	80. 2	111. 4	142. 1	173. 2	204. 1	235. 2	266. 3
19. 2	50. 1	81. 2	112. 4	143. 3	174. 4	205. 3	236. 1	267. 2
20. 4	51. 2	82. 1	113. 4	144. 1	175. 2	206. 3	237. 4	268. 3
21. 4	52. 2	83. 3	114. 2	145. 3	176. 2	207. 4	238. 3	269. 4
22. 1	53. 1	84. 3	115. 1	146. 1	177. 1	208. 3	239. 2	270. 2
23. 1	54. 1	85. 1	116. 2	147. 1	178. 1	209. 3	240. 4	271. 1
24. 1	55. 3	86. 3	117. 3	148. 2	179. 4	210. 2	241. 1	272. 1
25. 3	56. 3	87. 3	118. 4	149. 2	180. 1	211. 2	242. 3	273. 4
26. 1	57. 2	88. 3	119. 1	150. 3	181. 2	212. 4	243. 3	274. 3
27. 1	58. 4	89. 4	120. 1	151. 1	182. 3	213. 3	244. 3	275. 3
28. 3	59. 1	90. 4	121. 1	152. 1	183. 2	214. 4	245. 3	276. 2
29. 2	60. 4	91. 3	122. 3	153. 2	184. 3	215. 4	246. 3	
30. 1	61. 3	92. 2	123. 3	154. 3	185. 2	216. 4	247. 3	
31. 3	62. 1	93. 4	124. 3	155. 1	186. 1	217. 2	248. 2	

2. NAB DOMAIN: HUMAN RESOURCES

UNDERSTANDING THE DEPARTMENTS AND MANAGING HUMAN RESOURCES

1. *1*	17. *4*	33. *1*	49. *2*	65. *1*	81. *4*	97. *1*	113. *1*	129. *2*
2. *2*	18. *4*	34. *4*	50. *4*	66. *4*	82. *4*	98. *2*	114. *3*	130. *4*
3. *1*	19. *1*	35. *3*	51. *1*	67. *2*	83. *3*	99. *4*	115. *1*	131. *3*
4. *4*	20. *1*	36. *2*	52. *3*	68. *1*	84. *4*	100. *4*	116. *3*	132. *4*
5. *3*	21. *2*	37. *3*	53. *1*	69. *2*	85. *4*	101. *1*	117. *4*	133. *3*
6. *3*	22. *3*	38. *1*	54. *1*	70. *1*	86. *3*	102. *1*	118. *4*	134. *2*
7. *4*	23. *4*	39. *3*	55. *4*	71. *4*	87. *3*	103. *2*	119. *1*	135. *4*
8. *4*	24. *3*	40. *4*	56. *4*	72. *2*	88. *4*	104. *1*	120. *4*	136. *2*
9. *4*	25. *3*	41. *3*	57. *4*	73. *4*	89. *4*	105. *3*	121. *4*	137. *4*
10. *4*	26. *4*	42. *3*	58. *1*	74. *3*	90. *4*	106. *4*	122. *3*	138. *4*
11. *3*	27. *2*	43. *2*	59. *1*	75. *3*	91. *4*	107. *3*	123. *4*	139. *1*
12. *1*	28. *1*	44. *3*	60. *1*	76. *2*	92. *4*	108. *4*	124. *4*	
13. *1*	29. *1*	45. *3*	61. *1*	77. *1*	93. *3*	109. *3*	125. *2*	
14. *2*	30. *4*	46. *3*	62. *2*	78. *3*	94. *4*	110. *4*	126. *3*	
15. *1*	31. *3*	47. *3*	63. *1*	79. *3*	95. *2*	111. *3*	127. *2*	
16. *1*	32. *3*	48. *2*	64. *1*	80. *4*	96. *2*	112. *3*	128. *4*	

3. NAB DOMAIN: FINANCE/BUSINESS

LEARNING TO MANAGE THE ORGANIZATION'S FINANCES

1. *2*	13. *1*	25. *1*	37. *3*	49. *3*	61. *4*	73. *1*	85. *2*	97. *1*
2. *3*	14. *3*	26. *3*	38. *2*	50. *3*	62. *2*	74. *2*	86. *3*	98. *1*
3. *1*	15. *1*	27. *2*	39. *1*	51. *1*	63. *2*	75. *2*	87. *2*	99. *4*
4. *4*	16. *1*	28. *4*	40. *2*	52. *2*	64. *3*	76. *3*	88. *3*	100. *4*
5. *1*	17. *1*	29. *2*	41. *1*	53. *4*	65. *1*	77. *3*	89. *3*	101. *4*
6. *2*	18. *3*	30. *1*	42. *2*	54. *1*	66. *2*	78. *2*	90. *2*	
7. *2*	19. *2*	31. *4*	43. *1*	55. *1*	67. *3*	79. *2*	91. *3*	
8. *4*	20. *4*	32. *2*	44. *2*	56. *3*	68. *2*	80. *1*	92. *3*	
9. *3*	21. *3*	33. *4*	45. *2*	57. *3*	69. *1*	81. *4*	93. *4*	
10. *2*	22. *1*	34. *1*	46. *2*	58. *1*	70. *2*	82. *2*	94. *3*	
11. *1*	23. *3*	35. *3*	47. *1*	59. *3*	71. *1*	83. *1*	95. *3*	
12. *2*	24. *4*	36. *1*	48. *3*	60. *3*	72. *2*	84. *3*	96. *2*	

LEGAL AND BUSINESS TERMINOLOGY

1. 4	5. 2	9. 2	13. 1	17. 2	21. 1	25. 4	29. 4	33. 2
2. 2	6. 1	10. 1	14. 2	18. 1	22. 2	26. 4	30. 1	34. 4
3. 1	7. 3	11. 2	15. 1	19. 3	23. 1	27. 1	31. 1	
4. 4	8. 1	12. 2	16. 1	20. 1	24. 2	28. 3	32. 1	

4. NAB DOMAIN: ENVIRONMENT

LEARNING THE CONTINUUM OF LONG-TERM CARE

1. 2	5. 4
2. 2	6. 2
3. 4	7. 2
4. 2	8. 2

REGULATIONS

1. 1	9. 4	17. 1	25. 1	33. 3	41. 2	49. 2	57. 1	65. 2
2. 4	10. 4	18. 3	26. 1	34. 2	42. 1	50. 1	58. 3	66. 3
3. 2	11. 3	19. 1	27. 2	35. 4	43. 4	51. 1	59. 2	67. 1
4. 2	12. 3	20. 2	28. 1	36. 2	44. 3	52. 2	60. 4	68. 3
5. 1	13. 1	21. 1	29. 4	37. 3	45. 1	53. 4	61. 3	69. 4
6. 4	14. 4	22. 2	30. 1	38. 1	46. 1	54. 4	62. 2	70. 1
7. 3	15. 4	23. 2	31. 1	39. 1	47. 2	55. 1	63. 4	
8. 2	16. 3	24. 4	32. 4	40. 3	48. 4	56. 1	64. 2	

5. NAB DOMAIN: PATIENT/RESIDENT CARE

THE AGING PROCESS: OVERVIEW AND THEORIES

1. 2	4. 1
2. 2	5. 1
3. 4	6. 1

MEDICAL AND RELATED TERMS: SPECIALIZATIONS

1. 3	5. 3	9. 1	13. 2
2. 4	6. 2	10. 1	14. 1
3. 4	7. 3	11. 3	15. 2
4. 3	8. 1	12. 2	

MEDICATIONS/THERAPEUTIC ACTIONS OF DRUGS

1. 2	5. 1	9. 1	13. 3
2. 1	6. 4	10. 4	14. 4
3. 1	7. 4	11. 2	15. 2
4. 1	8. 3	12. 4	16. 2

ABBREVIATIONS

1. 1	5. 4	9. 1	13. 2	17. 1	21. 2	25. 3	29. 3	33. 2
2. 2	6. 1	10. 1	14. 3	18. 3	22. 1	26. 1	30. 1	34. 3
3. 2	7. 3	11. 1	15. 2	19. 1	23. 4	27. 2	31. 1	
4. 4	8. 4	12. 3	16. 4	20. 3	24. 2	28. 3	32. 4	

PREFIXES

1. 1	7. 2	13. 1	19. 4	25. 1	31. 2	37. 3	43. 3	49. 2
2. 1	8. 4	14. 4	20. 4	26. 4	32. 1	38. 1	44. 1	50. 1
3. 4	9. 2	15. 4	21. 1	27. 2	33. 2	39. 4	45. 1	
4. 2	10. 4	16. 3	22. 1	28. 2	34. 1	40. 2	46. 1	
5. 1	11. 2	17. 1	23. 1	29. 3	35. 4	41. 2	47. 3	
6. 4	12. 4	18. 1	24. 2	30. 3	36. 1	42. 2	48. 2	

SUFFIXES

1. 3	5. 3	9. 2	13. 1	17. 4	21. 2
2. 4	6. 2	10. 1	14. 2	18. 3	22. 3
3. 4	7. 4	11. 1	15. 2	19. 1	23. 2
4. 4	8. 4	12. 4	16. 4	20. 1	

DISEASES

1. 4	9. 2	17. 2	25. 3	33. 3	41. 4	49. 1	57. 3
2. 3	10. 3	18. 3	26. 3	34. 2	42. 2	50. 3	58. 2
3. 1	11. 3	19. 2	27. 1	35. 1	43. 1	51. 1	59. 2
4. 4	12. 1	20. 2	28. 4	36. 2	44. 2	52. 3	60. 1
5. 1	13. 1	21. 1	29. 4	37. 4	45. 1	53. 3	61. 4
6. 4	14. 2	22. 2	30. 1	38. 2	46. 4	54. 3	62. 3
7. 2	15. 4	23. 4	31. 1	39. 2	47. 1	55. 1	63. 3
8. 2	16. 2	24. 1	32. 4	40. 4	48. 1	56. 4	64. 3

6. FACILITY POLICIES

PUTTING THE SYSTEMS TOGETHER

1. 2	21. 1	41. 3	61. 3	81. 3	101. 2	121. 4	141. 3	161. 4
2. 3	22. 3	42. 4	62. 4	82. 3	102. 1	122. 2	142. 4	162. 3
3. 2	23. 1	43. 3	63. 2	83. 1	103. 4	123. 4	143. 3	163. 1
4. 4	24. 1	44. 2	64. 2	84. 3	104. 4	124. 4	144. 3	164. 3
5. 2	25. 3	45. 1	65. 2	85. 1	105. 3	125. 4	145. 3	165. 3
6. 4	26. 3	46. 2	66. 2	86. 3	106. 2	126. 3	146. 2	166. 1
7. 1	27. 2	47. 4	67. 2	87. 3	107. 3	127. 4	147. 4	167. 3
8. 3	28. 4	48. 2	68. 1	88. 2	108. 1	128. 2	148. 3	168. 1
9. 1	29. 4	49. 4	69. 4	89. 4	109. 1	129. 1	149. 1	169. 1
10. 3	30. 2	50. 4	70. 1	90. 4	110. 1	130. 3	150. 4	170. 2
11. 4	31. 2	51. 3	71. 1	91. 4	111. 2	131. 1	151. 4	171. 4
12. 3	32. 4	52. 3	72. 3	92. 3	112. 2	132. 2	152. 2	172. 3
13. 3	33. 2	53. 2	73. 3	93. 1	113. 4	133. 4	153. 4	173. 3
14. 2	34. 3	54. 3	74. 1	94. 2	114. 4	134. 3	154. 3	
15. 4	35. 4	55. 3	75. 2	95. 4	115. 3	135. 4	155. 2	
16. 4	36. 1	56. 2	76. 2	96. 3	116. 3	136. 3	156. 2	
17. 1	37. 4	57. 2	77. 2	97. 2	117. 3	137. 2	157. 3	
18. 2	38. 2	58. 1	78. 3	98. 3	118. 3	138. 3	158. 4	
19. 2	39. 1	59. 3	79. 4	99. 2	119. 2	139. 3	159. 3	
20. 2	40. 4	60. 1	80. 1	100. 4	120. 1	140. 1	160. 4